CASE REVIEW
Cardiac Imaging

Series Editor

David M. Yousem, MD, MBA
Professor of Radiology
Director of Neuroradiology
Russell H. Morgan Department of Radiology and Radiological Science
The Johns Hopkins Medical Institutions
Baltimore, Maryland

Other Volumes in the CASE REVIEW Series

- Brain Imaging
- Breast Imaging
- Emergency Radiology
- Gastrointestinal Imaging
- General and Vascular Ultrasound
- Genitourinary Imaging
- Head and Neck Imaging
- Musculoskeletal Imaging
- Nuclear Medicine
- OB/GYN Ultrasound
- Pediatric Imaging
- Spine Imaging
- Thoracic Imaging
- Vascular and Interventional Imaging

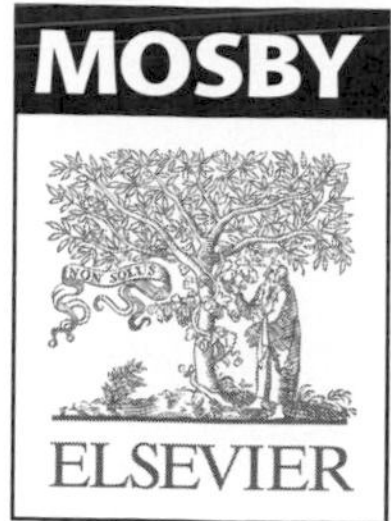

Gautham P. Reddy, MD, MPH
Associate Professor of Radiology
Director, Diagnostic Radiology Residency Program
Chief, Cardiac Imaging
Chief, Cardiac and Pulmonary Imaging
(VA Medical Center)
University of California, San Francisco
San Francisco, California

Robert M. Steiner, MD
Professor of Radiology
Director, Thoracic Radiology
Temple University Hospital
Clinical Professor of Radiology
The University of Pennsylvania School of Medicine
Philadelphia, Pennsylvania

WITH 217 ILLUSTRATIONS

CASE REVIEW

Cardiac Imaging

CASE REVIEW SERIES

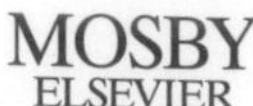

1600 John F. Kennedy Blvd.
Suite 1800
Philadelphia, PA 19103-2899

CARDIAC IMAGING: CASE REVIEW

Copyright © 2006, Elsevier Inc. All rights reserved.

No part of this publication may be reproduced or transmitted in any form or by any means, electronic or mechanical, including photocopying, recording, or any information storage and retrieval system, without permission in writing from the publisher.
Permissions may be sought directly from Elsevier's Health Sciences Rights Department in Philadelphia, PA, USA: phone: (+1) 215 239 3804, fax: (+1) 215 239 3805, e-mail: healthpermissions@elsevier.com. You may also complete your request on-line via the Elsevier homepage (http://www.elsevier.com), by selecting 'Customer Support' and then 'Obtaining Permissions'.

NOTICE

Knowledge and best practice in this field are constantly changing. As new research and experience broaden our knowledge, changes in practice, treatment and drug therapy may become necessary or appropriate. Readers are advised to check the most current information provided (i) on procedures featured or (ii) by the manufacturer of each product to be administered, to verify the recommended dose or formula, the method and duration of administration, and contraindications. It is the responsibility of the practitioner, relying on their own experience and knowledge of the patient, to make diagnoses, to determine dosages and the best treatment for each individual patient, and to take all appropriate safety precautions. To the fullest extent of the law, neither the Publisher nor the Editors assume any liability for any injury and/or damage to persons or property arising out or related to any use of the material contained in this book.

Library of Congress Cataloging-in-Publication Data

Reddy, Gautham P.
Cardiac imaging / Gautham P. Reddy, Robert M. Steiner — 1st ed.
p. ; cm. — (Case review series)
ISBN-13: 978-0-323-01176-1 ISBN-10: 0-323-01176-4
1. Heart—Imaging.
[DNLM: 1. Cardiovascular Diseases—radiography—Case Reports.
2. Diagnostic Imaging—methods—Case Reports. WG 141.5.R2 R313c 2006]
I. Steiner, Robert M. II. Title. III. Series.
RC683.5.142R43 2006
616.1'20757—dc22 2005054402

Acquisitions Editor: Meghan McAteer
Editorial Assistant: Elizabeth Schweizer

ISBN-13 978 0 323 01176-1
ISBN-10 0-323 01176-4

Printed in the United States of America.

Last digit is the print number: 9 8 7 6 5 4 3 2

Working together to grow
libraries in developing countries
www.elsevier.com | www.bookaid.org | www.sabre.org
ELSEVIER BOOK AID International Sabre Foundation

To Gayatri, Maurya, and Kanishka
GPR

To Marilyn, Emily, Peter, and Sophia
RMS

My experience in teaching medical students, residents, fellows, practicing radiologists, and clinicians has been that they love the case conference format more than any other approach. I hope that the reason for this is not a reflection on my lecturing ability, but rather that people stay awake, alert, and on their toes more when they are in the hot seat (or may be the next person to assume the hot seat). In the dozens of continuing medical education courses I have directed, the case review sessions are almost always the most popular parts of the courses.

The idea of this Case Review series grew out of a need for books designed as exam preparation tools for the resident, fellow, or practicing radiologist about to take the boards or the certificate of additional qualification (CAQ) exams. Anxiety runs extremely high concerning the content of these exams, administered as unknown cases. Residents, fellows, and practicing radiologists are very hungry for formats that mimic this exam setting and that cover the types of cases they will encounter and have to accurately describe. In addition, books of this ilk serve as excellent practical reviews of a field and can help a practicing board-certified radiologist keep his or her skills sharpened. Thus heads banged together, and Mosby and I arrived at the format of the volume herein, which is applied consistently to each volume in the series. We believe that these volumes will strengthen the ability of the reader to interpret studies. By formatting the individual cases so that they can "stand alone," these case review books can be read in a leisurely fashion, a case at a time, on the whim of the reader.

The content of each volume is organized into three sections based on difficulty of interpretation and/or the rarity of the lesion presented. There are the Opening Round cases, which graduating radiology residents should have relatively little difficulty mastering. The Fair Game section consists of cases that require more study, but most people should get into the ballpark with their differential diagnoses. Finally, there is the Challenge section. Most fellows or fellowship-trained practicing radiologists will be able to mention entities in the differential diagnoses of these challenging cases, but one shouldn't expect to consistently "hit home runs" à la Mark McGwire. The Challenge cases are really designed to whet one's appetite for further reading on these entities and to test one's wits. Within each of these sections, the selection of cases is entirely random, as one would expect at the boards (in your office or in Louisville).

For many cases in this series, a specific diagnosis may not be what is expected—the quality of the differential diagnosis and the inclusion of appropriate options are most important. Teaching how to distinguish between the diagnostic options (taught in the question and answer and comment sections) will be the goal of the authors of each Case Review volume.

The best way to go through these books is to look at the images, guess the diagnosis, answer the questions, and then turn the page for the answers. If there are two cases on a page, do them two at a time. No peeking!

Mosby (through the strong work of Liz Corra) and I have recruited most of the authors of THE REQUISITES series (editor, James Thrall, MD) to create Case Review books for their subspecialties. To meet the needs of certain subspecialties and to keep each of the volumes to a consistent, practical size, some specialties will have more than one volume (e.g., ultrasound, interventional and vascular radiology, and neuroradiology). Nonetheless, the pleasing tone of THE REQUISITES series and its emphasis on condensing the fields of radiology into its foundations will be inculcated into the Case Review volumes. In many situations, THE REQUISITES authors have enlisted new coauthors to breathe a novel approach and excitement into the cases submitted. I think the fact that so many of THE REQUISITES authors are "on board" for this new series is a testament to their dedication to teaching. I hope that the success of THE REQUISITES is duplicated with the new Case Review series. Just as THE REQUISITES series provides coverage of the essentials in each subspecialty and successfully meets that overwhelming need in the market, I hope that the Case Review series successfully meets the overwhelming need in the market for practical, focused case reviews.

David M. Yousem, MD, MBA

The latest Case Review edition, *Cardiac Imaging* by Gautham Reddy and Robert Steiner, is quite timely. Coronary artery CT angiography is moving from a research technique to the clinical arena and even in some cases to the Emergency Department. Radiologists must become well versed with this anatomy or they may see this technique vanish before their eyes into the cardiologists' sphere of influence. At the same time, cardiac MRI is becoming even more widely employed in a number of morphologic and physiologic studies that compete with traditional nuclear medicine techniques. I believe that radiology must maintain the lead in developing new applications and innovative invasive procedures to continue to lead the cardiac/cardiovascular field. This means that we all must learn the anatomy and pathology as well as our clinical colleagues.

Drs. Reddy and Steiner have compiled a wonderful array of cases that demonstrate the power of various modalities in our imaging armamentarium. At the same time they cover the wide variety of diseases that may affect children and adults with cardiovascular pathology. I believe that this will be the most challenging, but also a very valuable resource for trainees and cardiac imagers from all walks of medicine. I congratulate the authors on their hard work.

The philosophy of the Case Review series is to review each specialty in a challenging and interactive way. Each book in the series has gradations of difficulty so that the reader can assess his or her proficiency and can use this self-evaluation to guide continued education. Since each case in the book is distinct, this is the kind of text that can be picked up and read at any time in your day, in your career.

I am very pleased to welcome the *Cardiac Imaging: Case Review* edition to the ever-growing Case Review family.

David M. Yousem, MD, MBA
Case Review Series Editor

Michael B. Gotway, MD
Scottsdale Medical Imaging, An Affiliate of Southwestern Diagnostic Imaging, Ltd.
Scottsdale, Arizona
Clinical Associate Professor, Diagnostic Radiology and Pulmonary/Critical Care Medicine
University of California, San Francisco
Department of Radiology
San Francisco, California

Charles B. Higgins, MD
Professor of Radiology
University of California, San Francisco
San Francisco, California

Karen G. Ordovas, MD
Fellow
Department of Radiology
University of California, San Francisco
San Francisco, California

Shalini Veerareddy, MD
Consultant Radiologist
Apollo Hospital
Hyderabad, India

Mei-Han Wu, MD
Staff Radiologist
Taipei Veterans General Hospital
Taipei, Taiwan

Our goal in writing *Cardiac Imaging: Case Review* was to provide a case-based learning guide and review in cardiovascular radiology for the resident or practicing radiologist. This book may be used in preparation for the American Board of Radiology's new "virtual" cardiac imaging component of the oral examination in diagnostic radiology. Moreover, this volume may have particular value because of new technological developments and the current emphasis on cardiac imaging among radiologists and cardiologists.

We have tried to include a broad range of cardiovascular pathology, much of which will be encountered frequently in a busy clinical practice. Some of the cases are more unusual but have been included because they raise important teaching points or because the imaging findings are characteristic and are essential to establishing the diagnosis.

The cases may include conventional radiographs, CT, or MRI; some cases incorporate more than one modality. Advanced techniques such as delayed-enhancement MRI, velocity-encoded cine MRI, and CT angiography are included.

The book is divided into three sections: Opening Round contains cases that are relatively straightforward. Fair Game consists of cases that may require further thought or analysis. The last section, Challenge, comprises cases that are more difficult because of their complex imaging findings, advanced techniques, or rarity.

We hope that the reader finds this book to be an easy-to-read review of cardiac imaging.

Gautham P. Reddy, MD
Robert M. Steiner, MD

Opening Round 1

Fair Game 47

Challenge 127

Index of Cases 173

Index of Terms 175

Opening Round

CASE 1

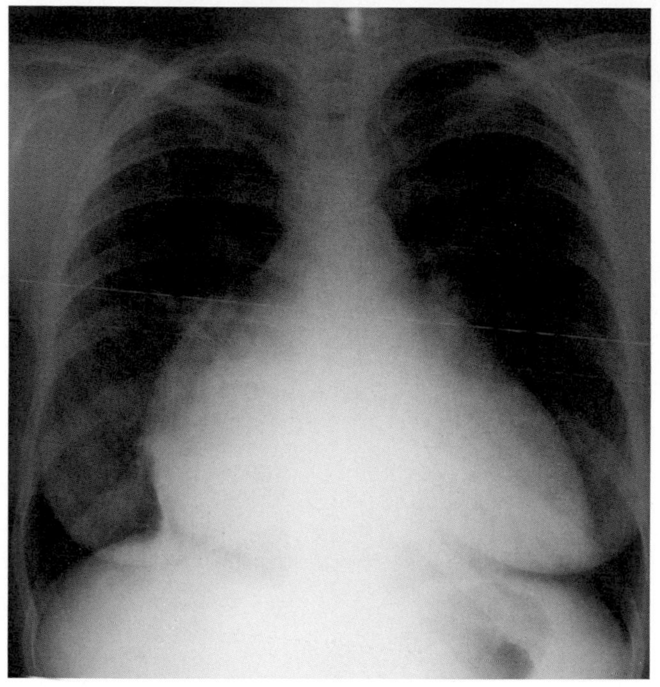

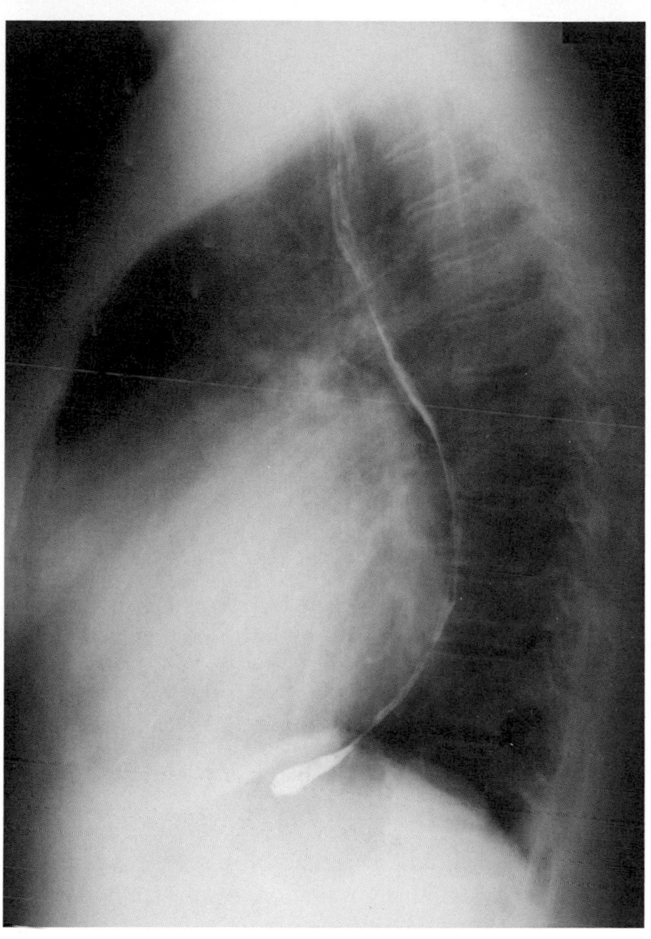

1. Which chamber(s) are enlarged?
2. What is the most likely diagnosis?
3. What is the most common cause of papillary muscle rupture?
4. What is the major valve lesion in acute rheumatic fever?

ANSWERS

CASE 1

Mitral Regurgitation

1. Left atrium and left ventricle.
2. Mitral regurgitation.
3. Myocardial ischemia or infarction.
4. Mitral regurgitation.

Reference

Bonow RO, Cheitlin MD, Crawford MH, Douglas PS. Task Force 3: valvular heart disease. *J Am Coll Cardiol* 45:1334–1340, 2005.

Cross-Reference

Cardiac Imaging: THE REQUISITES, 2nd edition, pp 180–184.

Comment

Mitral regurgitation is caused by a malfunction of any part of the mitral apparatus, including the valve leaflets, chordae, papillary muscles, mitral annulus, and the adjacent left ventricular wall. Causes of mitral regurgitation include ischemic cardiomyopathy, myocardial infarction, papillary muscle rupture, rheumatic heart disease, endocarditis, and trauma.

Chest radiographic findings of mitral regurgitation vary depending on the chronicity and severity of disease. Acute, severe mitral regurgitation results in pulmonary venous hypertension and alveolar edema without significant cardiac enlargement. After several days, the heart dilates and interstitial edema persists. After weeks to months, the left atrium and ventricle are enlarged, and the pulmonary pattern is variable.

Echocardiography is commonly used to grade the severity of mitral regurgitation. MRI can be used to quantify the regurgitant fraction.

Notes

Mitral Regurg Causes:
- ischemic cardiomyopathy
- MI
- Papillary muscle rupture
- Rheumatic Heart Dz
- Endocarditis

CASE 2

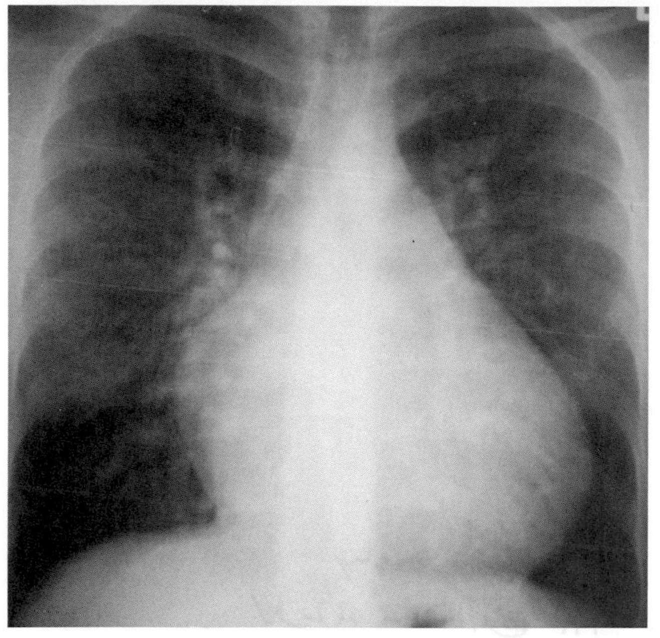

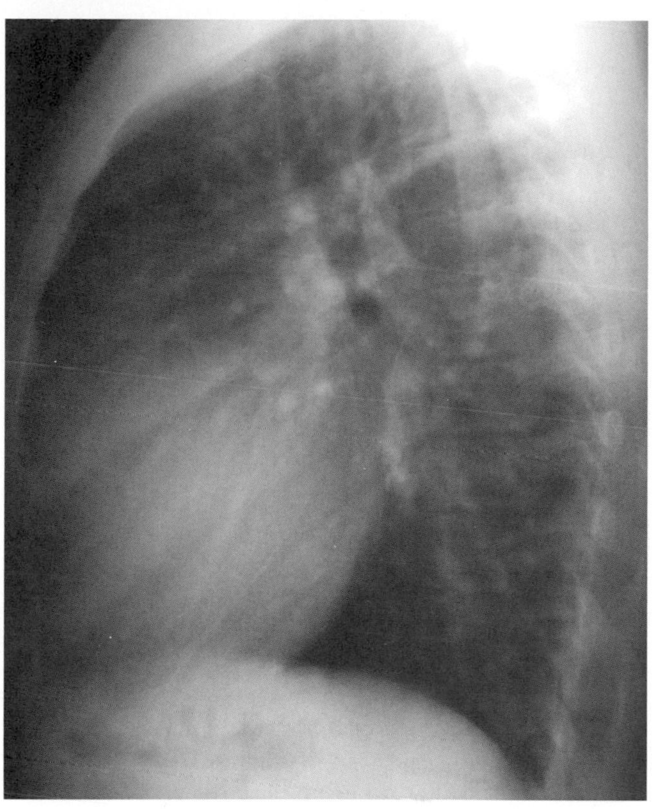

1. Is shunt vascularity present?
2. Is the left atrium enlarged?
3. This patient is acyanotic. What is the most likely diagnosis?
4. What is another atrial-level shunt that can have this appearance?

CASE 2

Atrial Septal Defect

1. Yes.
2. No.
3. Atrial septal defect.
4. Partial anomalous pulmonary venous connection.

Reference

Wu JC, Child JS. Common congenital heart disorders in adults. *Curr Probl Cardiol* 29:641–700, 2004.

Cross-Reference

Cardiac Imaging: THE REQUISITES, 2nd edition, pp 324–326.

Comment

The chest radiograph shows shunt vascularity with a normal-sized left atrium. In an acyanotic patient, the most likely diagnosis is atrial septal defect (ASD).

There are several types of ASD, including ostium secundum, ostium primum, and sinus venosus. Ostium secundum ASD is the most common type and is the most frequently diagnosed left-to-right shunt in adulthood. An ostium primum ASD is present in atrioventricular septal defect (formerly known as endocardial cushion defect). Sinus venosus ASD is associated with partial anomalous pulmonary venous connection.

Although the chest radiograph may be normal when the shunt is small, pulmonary vascularity is usually increased (shunt vascularity). Typically, the main pulmonary artery, peripheral pulmonary branches, right atrium, and right ventricule are enlarged. The left atrium is not enlarged, an important sign that differentiates an ASD from a ventricular septal defect or patent ductus arteriosus. Partial anomalous pulmonary venous connection is another atrial-level shunt that can mimic an ASD physiologically and can appear similar to ASD on a chest radiograph.

Echocardiography can delineate the size and location of the ASD. MRI can be performed if echocardiography does not demonstrate a suspected ASD.

↑ Pulm Vascularity
nl (L) Atrium + (L) V
↑ (R) A + ↑ (R) V

Notes

ASD #1 Type = Ostium Secundum – Holt Oram
↳ #1 L→R shunt in adults

- Ostium Primum = part of ECD – Down's

- Sinus Venosus Defect
  - @ entrance of SVC
  - ass'd c̄ PAPVR

CASE 3

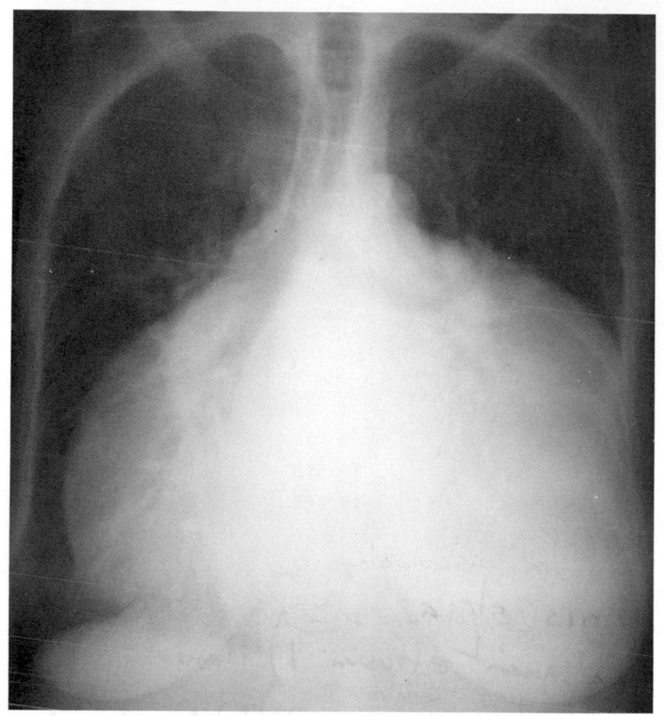

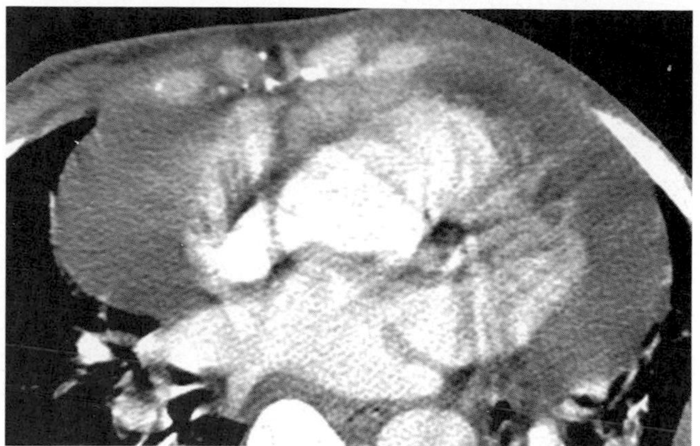

1. What is the differential diagnosis for a "wall-to-wall heart"?
2. What is the diagnosis?
3. Name two findings that suggest a malignant pericardial effusion.
4. What does pulsus paradoxus indicate?

CASE 3

Pericardial Effusion

1. Tricuspid regurgitation, dilated cardiomyopathy, pericardial effusion.
2. Pericardial effusion.
3. Nodularity of the pericardium, hemorrhagic effusion.
4. Cardiac tamponade.

Reference

Breen JF. Imaging of the pericardium. *J Thoracic Imaging* 16:47–54, 2001.

Cross-Reference

Cardiac Imaging: THE REQUISITES, 2nd edition, pp 203, 250–253.

Comment

The chest radiograph demonstrates massive enlargement of the cardiac silhouette ("wall-to-wall heart"). The CT scan shows a large pericardial effusion.

A small pericardial effusion is frequently not identified on chest radiography. As the pericardial effusion increases, the cardiac silhouette may acquire a globular ("water bottle") configuration, which results from obscuration of the normal bulges and indentations of the cardiac contours. Because a pericardial effusion can cause enlargement of the cardiac silhouette, it may be difficult to distinguish pericardial effusion from cardiomegaly on chest radiographs.

One differentiating feature is obscuration of the hilar vessels by a large pericardial effusion, which does not occur with cardiomegaly alone. Sometimes a pericardial effusion can cause an opaque band between the pericardial fat and the subpericardial fat on a lateral chest film, known as the "fat pad" sign. Although this sign is specific, its sensitivity for pericardial effusion is limited.

Echocardiography is more sensitive than plain films for the diagnosis of pericardial effusion. When a pericardial effusion is suggested by clinical or radiographic findings, echocardiography can confirm the diagnosis. CT and MRI also can demonstrate pericardial effusion and are useful for the identification of a hemorrhagic effusion and nodularity of the pericardium, both of which suggest a malignant effusion.

Signs of a malignant effusion: 1) Hemorrhagic 2) Nodularity of the pericardium

Pulsus Paradoxus = exaggerated drop in systolic BP during inspiration > 10 mm Hg

Indicates: - cardiac tamponade -or constrictive pericarditis

Notes

Wall-to Wall Heart DDx: - Pericardial Effusion
- Dilated Cardiomyopathy
- Tricuspid Regurgitation

Pulsus Paradoxus indicates: cardiac tamponade

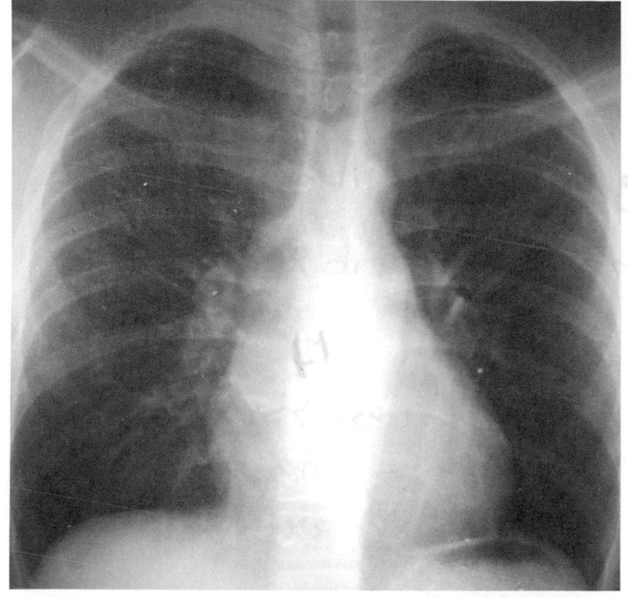

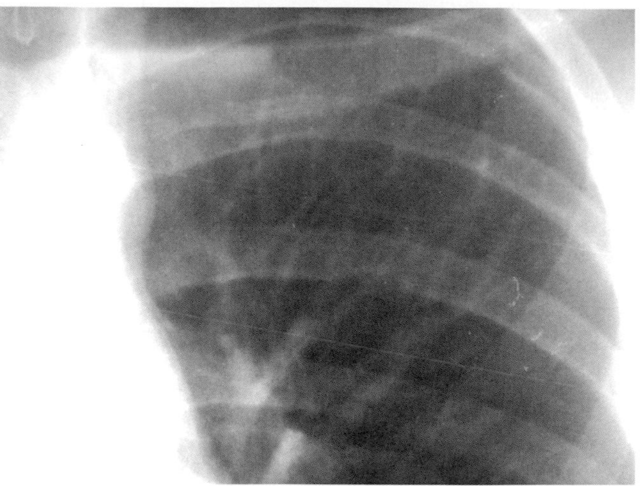

Close-up view of posteroanterior chest radiograph.

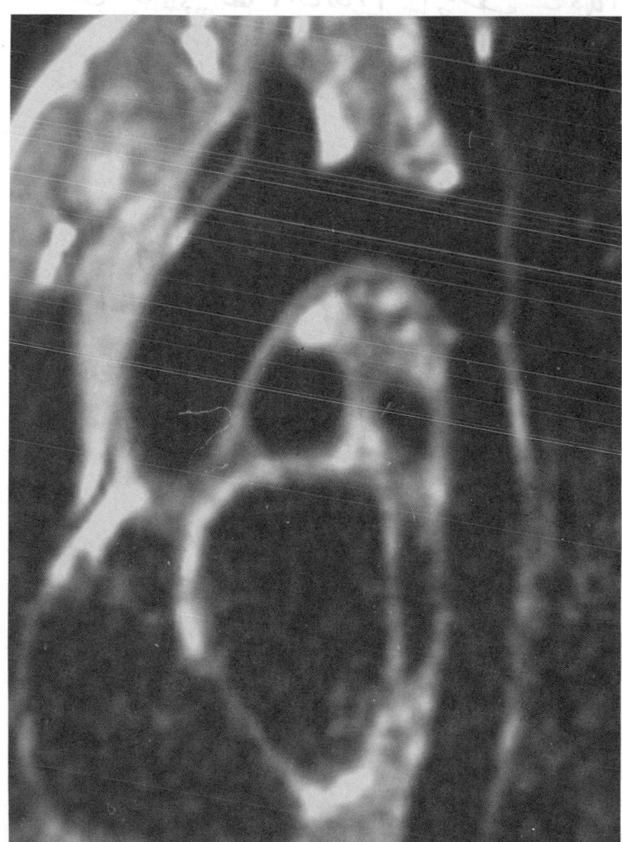

Oblique sagittal spin-echo MR image.

1. What sign describes the contour abnormality of the aorta?
2. Which rib abnormality is present?
3. What is the diagnosis?
4. Name four advantages of MRI over angiography for the diagnosis of this condition.

ANSWERS

CASE 4

Coarctation of the Aorta

1. "Figure 3" sign.
2. Rib notching.
3. Coarctation of the aorta.
4. Noninvasiveness, absence of ionizing radiation, lack of need for iodinated contrast agent, ability to measure collateral flow.

Reference

Reddy GP, Higgins CB. Magnetic resonance imaging of congenital heart disease: evaluation of morphology and function. *Semin Roentgenol* 38:342–351, 2003.

Cross-Reference

Cardiac Imaging: THE REQUISITES, 2nd edition, pp 414–422.

Comment

Infants may present with a preductal coarctation that results in congestive heart failure. Beyond infancy, a discrete juxtaductal coarctation is the most common type. Patients with a juxtaductal or postductal coarctation usually have hypertension or asymmetry of the upper extremity blood pressures on physical examination.

Chest radiographs may show a characteristic abnormal contour of the aortic arch, known as the "figure 3" sign, which is a double bulge just above and below the region of the aortic knob, as in this patient. Bilateral symmetrical rib notching can occur in an older child or adult.

MRI is now an important tool for the evaluation of coarctation of the aorta before and after surgical repair or balloon angioplasty. Because it is noninvasive and can provide complete anatomic and functional evaluation of coarctation, MRI can usually replace diagnostic angiography. MRI readily demonstrates narrowing of the aorta in patients with coarctation.

Notes

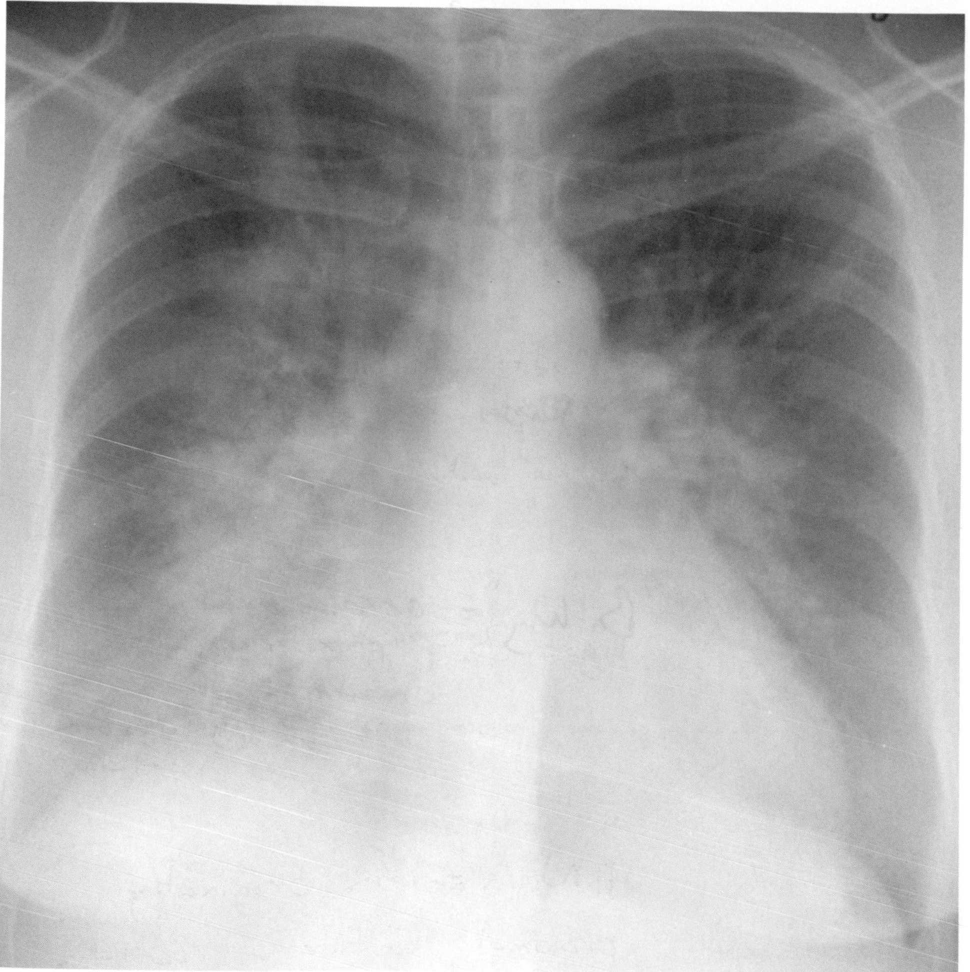

1. What is the distribution of the lung opacity?
2. What is the most likely diagnosis?
3. Name three radiographic features of pulmonary edema.
4. Name three radiographic features of congestive heart failure.

ANSWERS

CASE 5

Pulmonary Edema

1. Bilateral perihilar ("bat wing").
2. Pulmonary edema.
3. Kerley B lines, airspace opacity, and (in cardiogenic edema) enlarged pulmonary vessels.
4. Pulmonary edema, cardiomegaly, pleural effusions.

Reference

Morgan PW, Goodman LR. Pulmonary edema and adult respiratory distress syndrome. *Radiol Clin North Am* 29:943–963, 1991.

Cross-Reference

Cardiac Imaging: THE REQUISITES, 2nd edition, pp 27–32.

Comment

The chest radiograph demonstrates airspace opacities with peripheral sparing, known as the "bat wing" pattern, which is characteristic of cardiogenic pulmonary edema.

Pulmonary edema is related both to blood flow and blood pressure or to pressure alone. Elevation of pulmonary venous pressure can be secondary to left ventricular failure, mitral stenosis, and other causes of vascular obstruction distal to the pulmonary arterial bed. When pressure increases to between 12 and 18 mm Hg, pulmonary blood flow is redistributed to the upper lobes, which presents as enlargement of the upper lobe vessels ("cephalization") on chest radiographs. When pulmonary venous pressure rises above 18 mm Hg, pulmonary interstitial edema ensues. Kerley B lines—thin, horizontal, interlobular septal lines—are seen at the lung bases on chest radiographs. With elevation of pulmonary venous pressure above 25 mm Hg, alveolar edema develops, and chest radiographs may demonstrate opacities that involve the central portions of the lungs, sometimes producing a "bat wing" appearance.

If the pulmonary edema is related to congestive heart failure, the cardiac silhouette is enlarged, and pleural effusions are often seen on chest radiographs.

Notes

CASE 6

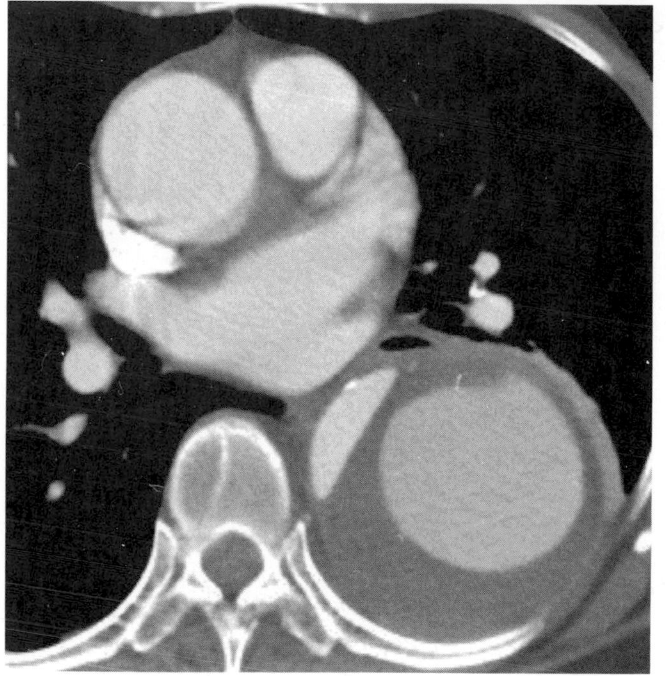

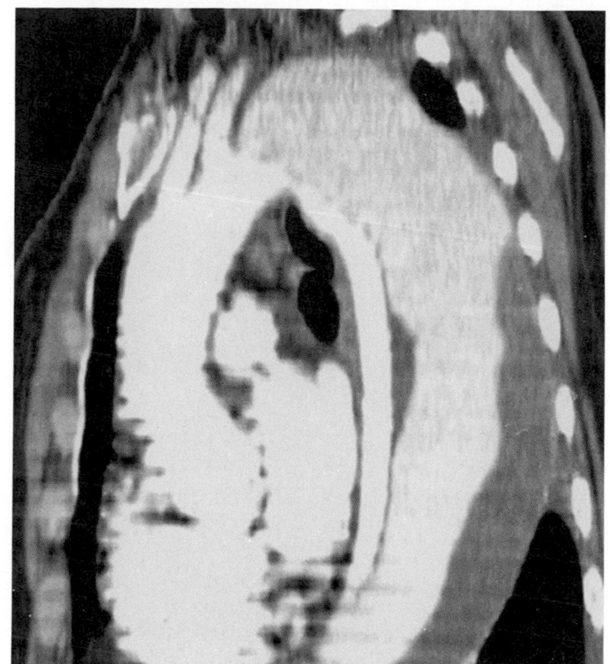

Multiplanar reformation of CT image

1. What is the diagnosis?
2. What is a Stanford type B dissection?
3. Name some important causes of aortic dissection.
4. Does this lesion require surgery?

CASE 7

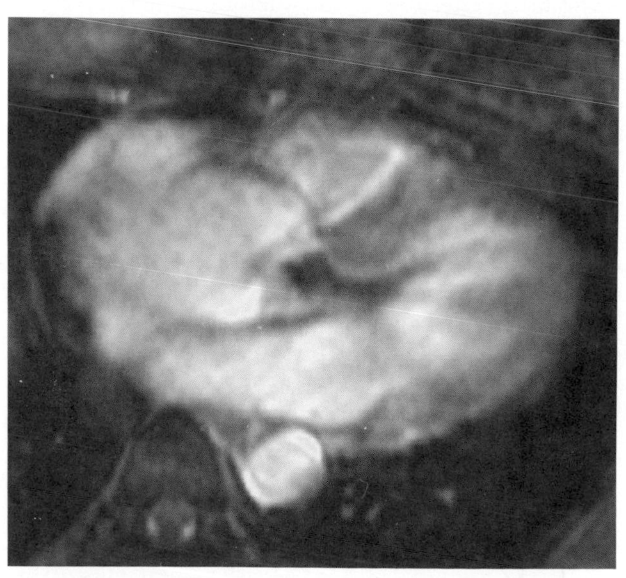

* Know the image

1. What is the diagnosis?
2. What MRI sequence is depicted?
3. What is the cause of this lesion in a patient with Marfan syndrome?
4. What other valve diseases are associated with Marfan syndrome?

CASE 6

Aortic Dissection, Stanford Type B

1. Aortic dissection, Stanford type B.
2. Dissection involving the descending aorta only, distal to the origin of the left subclavian artery.
3. Hypertension, annuloaortic ectasia, bicuspid aortic valve, aneurysm, vasculitis, trauma.
4. No.

Reference

Rubin GD. CT angiography of the thoracic aorta. *Semin Roentgenol* 38:115–134, 2003.

Cross-Reference

Cardiac Imaging: THE REQUISITES, 2nd edition, pp 371–380.

Comment

Aortic dissection is a separation of the aortic wall that results from intimal disruption. Blood can enter the aortic wall through a tear in the intima, extending proximally and distally in the media, displacing the intima inward. Typically blood flows in both the true and the false lumina, although the false channel is sometimes thrombosed.

The most common predisposing factor for aortic dissection is hypertension. Other etiologies include annuloaortic ectasia (which is associated with connective tissue disorders such as Marfan syndrome or Ehlers-Danlos syndrome), bicuspid aortic valve, aortic aneurysm, and arteritis.

Aortic dissection can be classified as Stanford type A (involving the ascending aorta) or type B (involving the descending aorta, distal to the left subclavian artery origin). The DeBakey classification system identifies three types of dissection: type I involves the ascending aorta and extends into the descending aorta; type II involves the ascending aorta only; and type III involves the descending aorta only, beyond the origin of the left subclavian artery.

CT has high accuracy for the diagnosis of aortic dissection. MRI has similar accuracy and can serve as an alternative imaging modality, especially when CT is contraindicated or in the setting of a chronic dissection. Transesophageal echocardiography can be useful but may have lower specificity than CT or MRI.

Notes

Aortic Dissection: Causes DDx: - HTN #1
- Annular Ectasia
  - Connective Tissue Disorder
    - Marfan's, Ehlers Danlos
- Bicuspid Valve
- Aneurysm
- Vasculitis

CASE 7

Aortic Regurgitation—Marfan Syndrome

1. Aortic regurgitation.
2. Cine-MRI.
3. Annuloaortic ectasia or leaflet prolapse.
4. Mitral and tricuspid valve prolapse, pulmonary regurgitation.

Reference

Bonow RO, Cheitlin MD, Crawford MH, Douglas PS. Task Force 3: valvular heart disease. *J Am Coll Cardiol* 45:1334–1340, 2005.

Cross-Reference

Cardiac Imaging: THE REQUISITES, 2nd edition, pp 169–174.

Comment

The cine-MR image demonstrates a flow jet emanating from the aortic valve into the left ventricle, indicating aortic regurgitation.

Marfan syndrome causes annuloaortic ectasia. Enlargement of the aortic annulus and prolapse of the valve leaflets can result in aortic regurgitation. Other complications of annuloaortic ectasia are dissection and aortic rupture. Marfan syndrome also is associated with prolapse of the mitral and tricuspid valves.

Chest radiographs demonstrate enlargement of the ascending aorta and left ventricle. Chronic, severe regurgitation can cause enlargement of the entire thoracic aorta. Pectus excavatum deformity and scoliosis may be present in patients with Marfan syndrome.

Echocardiography can be used to assess the degree of regurgitation. MRI is used to evaluate the size of the aorta and the extent of dilatation and to quantify the severity of regurgitation.

Patients with severe regurgitation require valve replacement. When the aorta is greater than 5 cm in diameter, valve surgery can be done in conjunction with graft replacement of the ascending aorta.

Notes

CASE 8

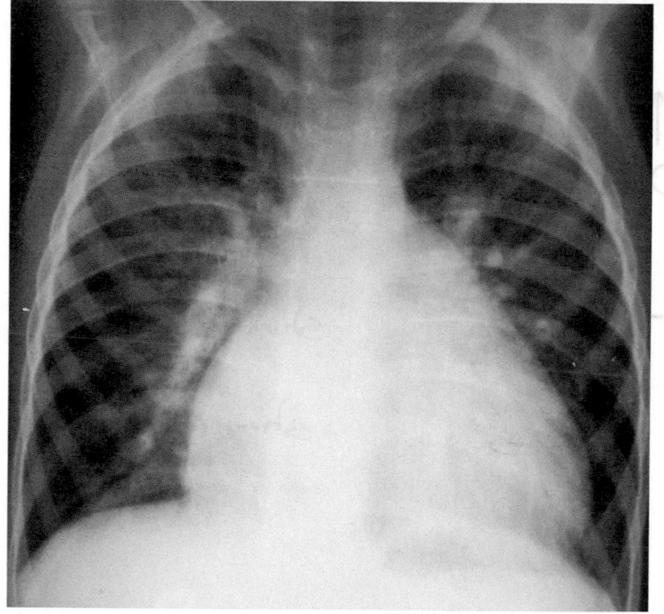

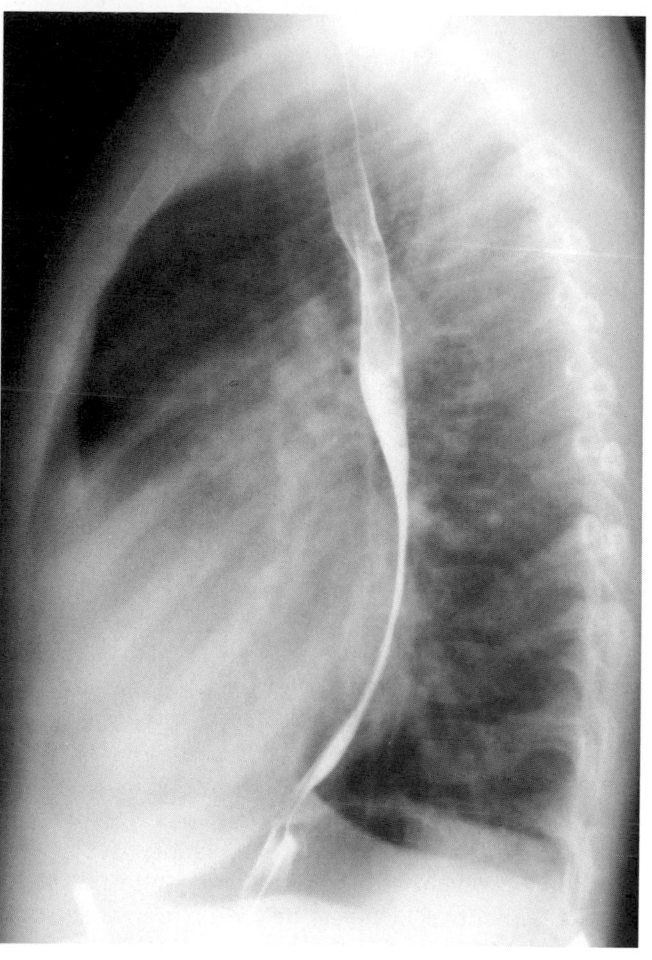

1. Is shunt vascularity present?
2. Is the left atrium enlarged?
3. Is the aortic arch enlarged?
4. In an acyanotic patient, what is the most likely diagnosis?

ANSWERS

CASE 8

Ventricular Septal Defect

1. Yes.
2. Yes.
3. No.
4. Ventricular septal defect.

Reference

Higgins CB. Radiography of congenital heart disease. In Webb WR, Higgins CB, editors: *Thoracic imaging: pulmonary and cardiovascular radiology*. Philadelphia, 2005, Lippincott Williams & Wilkins, pp 679–706.

Cross-Reference

Cardiac Imaging: THE REQUISITES, 2nd edition, pp 331–334.

Comment

The chest radiographs demonstrate cardiomegaly and shunt vascularity (increased vascularity). The left atrium is enlarged, signifying that the shunt is beyond the atrial level. The aortic knob is normal in size, indicating that the most likely lesion in an acyanotic patient is a ventricular septal defect (VSD). Patent ductus arteriosus typically causes dilation of the aortic knob.

If a VSD is small, the chest radiographs are usually normal. However, if the left-to-right shunt is large, shunt vascularity is identified on chest films, and the central pulmonary arteries, both ventricles, and the left atrium are enlarged.

Echocardiography usually demonstrates the location and size of the defect. MRI may be performed in certain patients to evaluate associated abnormalities or to define certain lesions such as a supracristal VSD, which may be difficult to image by echocardiography. Velocity-encoded cine phase–contrast MRI can be used to quantify the pulmonary-to-systemic flow ratio, which is an indicator of the severity of the shunt.

Notes

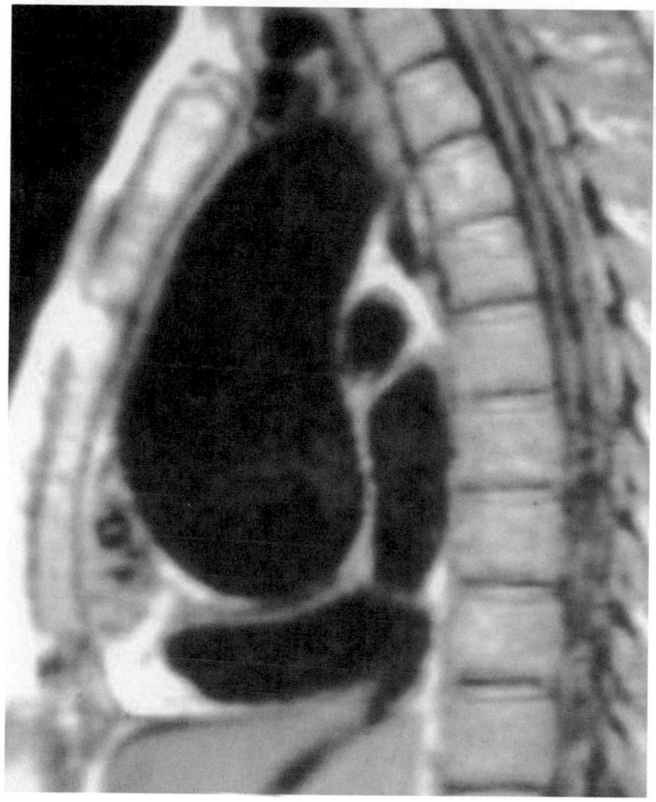
Sagittal spin-echo MR image.

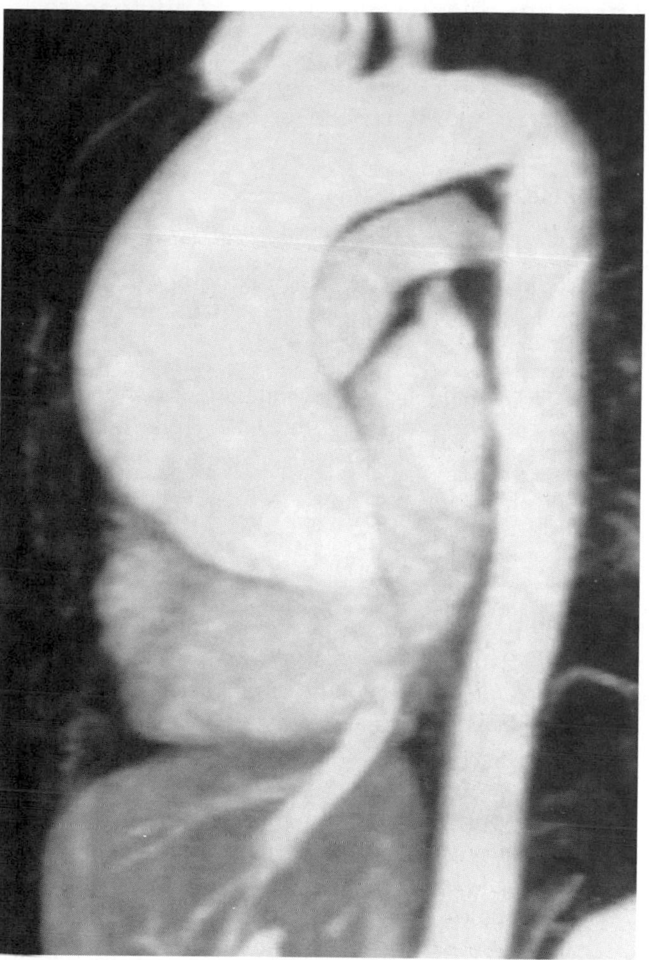
Maximum-intensity projection (MIP) of gadolinium-enhanced MR angiogram.

1. Which MRI sequences are shown?
2. What is the diagnosis?
3. Name two diseases that are associated with this condition.
4. Name three complications of this condition.

CASE 9

Aneurysm of Ascending Aorta—Annuloaortic Ectasia

1. Spin-echo (black blood) MRI and gadolinium-enhanced MRA (magnetic resonance angiogram, at right).
2. Annuloaortic ectasia.
3. Marfan syndrome and Ehlers-Danlos syndrome.
4. Aortic dissection, aortic rupture, aortic regurgitation.

3 complications
- Aortic Dissection
- Aortic Rupture
- Aortic Regurgitation

Reference

Reddy GP, Higgins CB. MR imaging of the thoracic aorta. *Magn Reson Imaging Clin N Am* 8:1–15, 2000.

Cross-Reference

Cardiac Imaging: THE REQUISITES, 2nd edition, pp 377, 380–382.

Comment

The MRI demonstrates enlargement of the aortic root and ascending aorta, which is characteristic of annuloaortic ectasia. The dilation of the aorta in this condition may stop at the sinotubular junction or extend to involve the entire ascending aorta, which is sometimes called the "tulip bulb" configuration. Annuloaortic ectasia results from cystic medial necrosis, which can be idiopathic or can be associated with Marfan syndrome or Ehlers-Danlos syndrome.

Complications of annuloaortic ectasia include aortic dissection, aortic rupture, and aortic regurgitation. Although 6 cm is the usual threshold of aortic diameter that necessitates surgery, operative repair may be indicated in annuloaortic ectasia when the aorta reaches a diameter of 5 cm owing to the high risk of rupture.

Notes

Annuloaortic Ectasia = dilated aortic root & ascending aorta
- appearance "Tulip bulb"
- DDx: - Connective Tissue Disorder
  - Marfan's
  - Ehlers-Danlos
  - Cystic Medial Necrosis - idiopathic

Complications: - Dissection
- Rupture
- Aortic Regurgitation

CASE 10

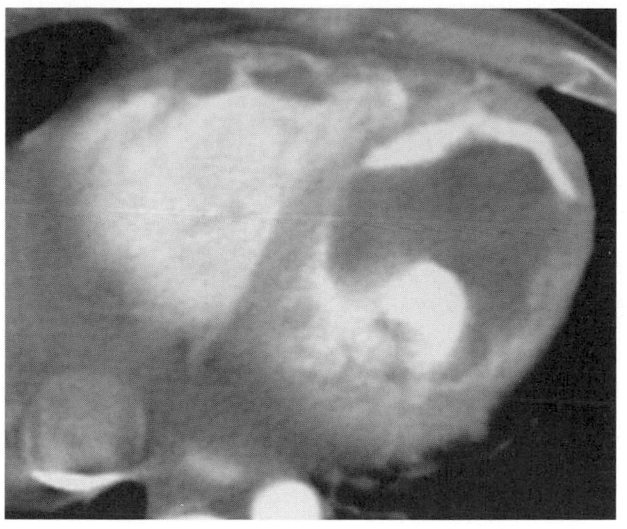

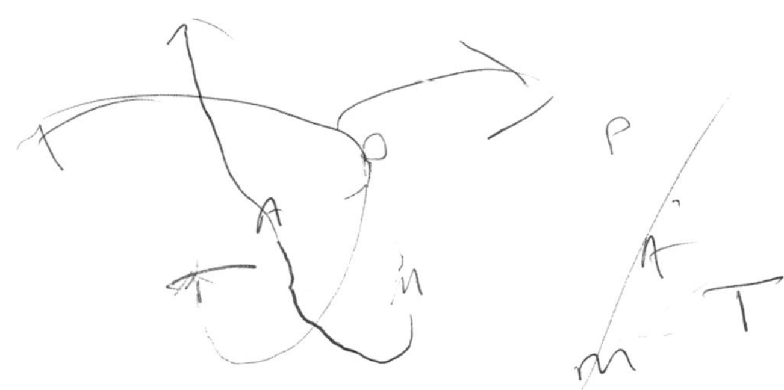

1. What is the most common mass in the heart?
2. Does this mass enhance?
3. What is the most likely diagnosis?
4. What imaging study is most specific for differentiating thrombus from neoplasm?

CASE 11

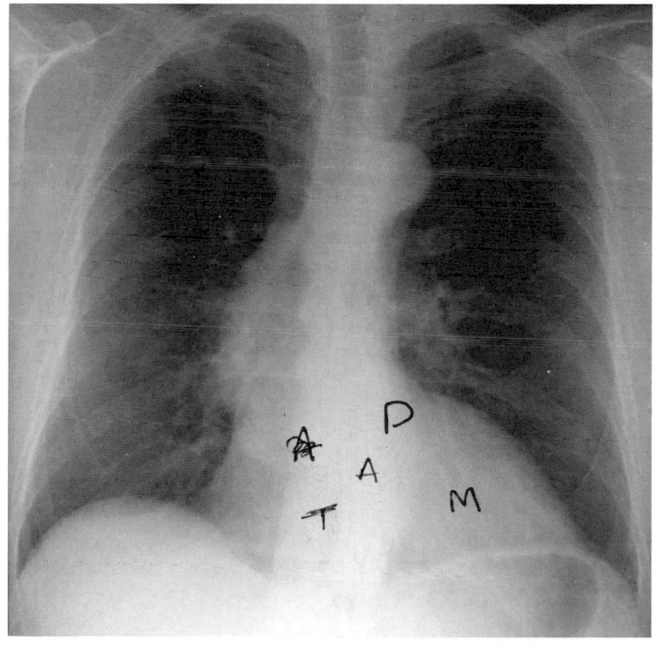

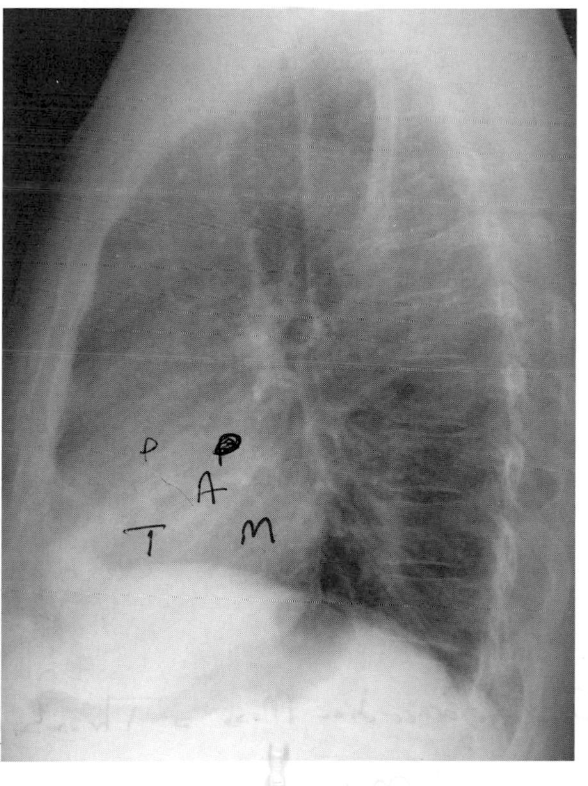

1. Which valve is abnormal?
2. What is the diagnosis?
3. What is the most common cause of this lesion?
4. If the peak velocity across the valve is 3 m/sec, what is the pressure gradient?

CASE 10

Left Ventricular Thrombus

1. Thrombus.
2. No.
3. Thrombus.
4. MRI.

Reference

Tatli S, Lipton MJ. CT for intracardiac thrombi and tumors. *Int J Cardiovasc Imaging* 21:115–131, 2005.

Cross-Reference

Cardiac Imaging: THE REQUISITES, 2nd edition, pp 268–270.

Comment

The contrast-enhanced CT scan shows a large, nonenhancing mass in the left ventricle. Although left ventricular thrombi are uncommon in the absence of a ventricular aneurysm, the lack of enhancement confirms that the mass is a thrombus. This patient had a coagulation disorder, and it was presumed that the thrombus developed in situ.

Thrombus is the most common cardiac or paracardiac mass. Among cardiac and paracardiac neoplasms, secondary tumors occur at 40 times the rate of primary neoplasms. Secondary tumors can involve the heart by direct extension (most commonly lymphoma or lymphadenopathy metastatic from lung or breast carcinoma) or by hematogenous spread (most commonly lung or breast carcinoma, melanoma). Primary benign tumors of the heart include myxoma, lipoma, and rhabdomyoma (associated with tuberous sclerosis). Primary malignant neoplasms include angiosarcoma and rhabdomyosarcoma.

MRI is the most accurate imaging examination for differentiation of tumor from thrombus. Neoplasms enhance homogeneously or heterogeneously after administration of gadolinium-chelate contrast agent, whereas thrombi do not enhance. On gradient-echo (GRE) MRI, tumor usually shows intermediate signal intensity, and thrombus tends to demonstrate low signal intensity. However, myxomas are often dark on GRE images.

Notes

#1 Cardiac/Paracardiac Mass = Thrombus

#1 Tumor = Met — Lung, Breast, Melanoma

Best Test = MRI

CASE 11

Aortic Stenosis

1. Aortic valve.
2. Aortic stenosis.
3. Bicuspid aortic valve.
4. 36 mm Hg.

Reference

Bonow RO, Cheitlin MD, Crawford MH, Douglas PS. Task Force 3: valvular heart disease. *J Am Coll Cardiol* 45:1334–1340, 2005.

Cross-Reference

Cardiac Imaging: THE REQUISITES, 2nd edition, pp 159–165.

Comment

The chest radiographs demonstrate calcification of the aortic valve, indicating valvular stenosis. The calcification is best demonstrated on the lateral view. The right side of the ascending aorta bulges secondary to poststenotic dilatation.

Isolated stenosis of the aortic valve is most commonly secondary to congenital bicuspid valve. Rheumatic heart disease is another important cause of aortic stenosis.

Mild-to-moderate aortic stenosis can cause left ventricular hypertrophy. The left ventricular border may be rounded or the cardiac apex may be elevated secondary to concentric left ventricular hypertrophy. More severe valvular stenosis can lead to enlargement of the left ventricle and atrium, as well as to hypertrophy. Owing to poststenotic dilatation, the ascending aortic contour bulges rightward. Calcification of the valve can develop as a result of degeneration and can be seen on CT or, when severe, on chest radiographs.

The pressure gradient across the valve can be calculated by use of the modified Bernoulli equation, $\Delta P = 4v^2$, where P is the pressure in mm Hg and v is peak velocity in m/sec. The peak velocity can be estimated by echocardiography or velocity-encoded cine phase contrast MRI.

Notes

PA: P, A, T, M

Lat View (Ant, Post): P, A, T, M

$\Delta P = 4v^2$

CASE 12

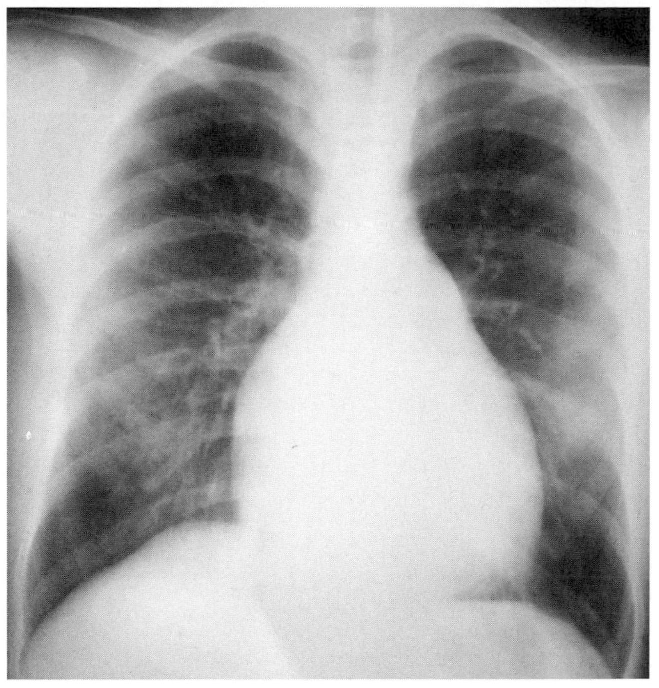

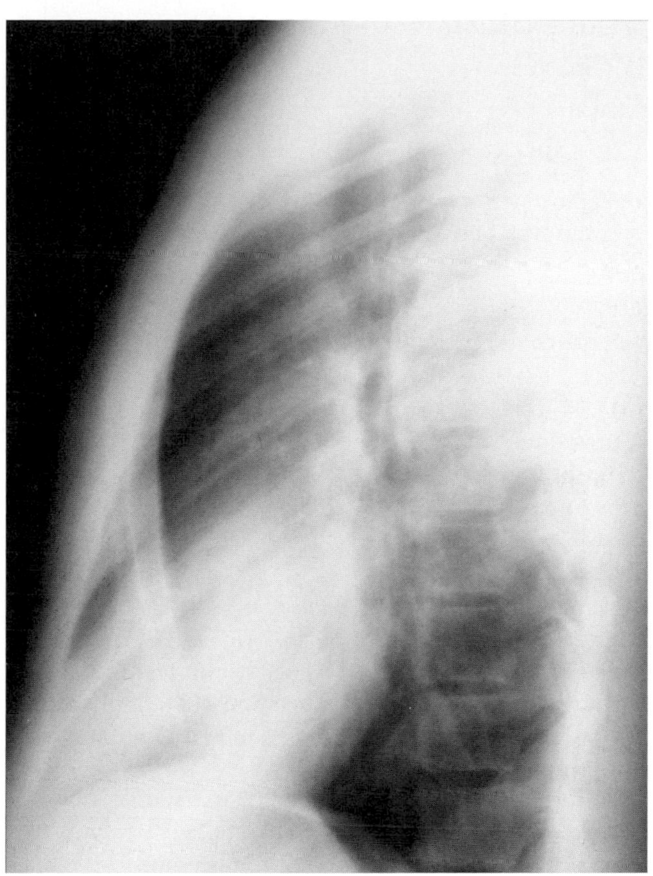

1. In which direction is the sternum displaced?
2. In which direction is the heart displaced?
3. What is the diagnosis?
4. Name at least one associated condition.

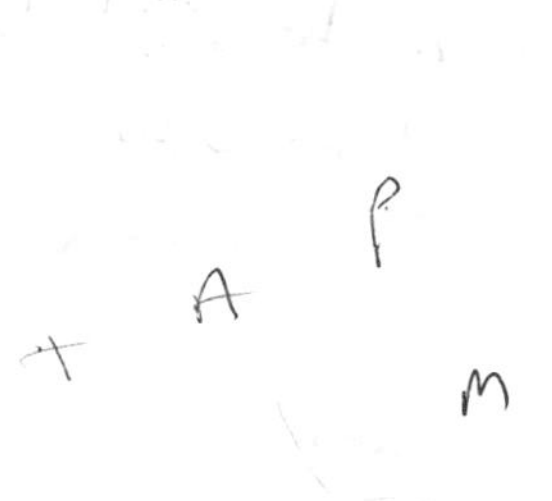

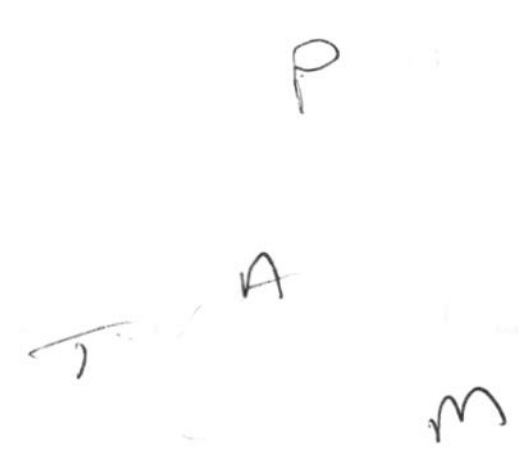

ANSWERS

CASE 12

Pectus Excavatum

1. Posteriorly.
2. To the left.
3. Pectus excavatum.
4. Marfan syndrome, Ehlers-Danlos syndrome, homocystinuria, Hunter-Hurler syndrome, mitral valve prolapse.

Reference

Ellis DG. Chest wall deformities in children. *Pediatr Ann* 18:161–165, 1989.

Cross-Reference

Cardiac Imaging: THE REQUISITES, 2nd edition, p 382.

Comment

The images demonstrate pectus excavatum, in which the sternum is displaced posteriorly and the heart is displaced to the left. Pectus excavatum is associated with a number of conditions, including Marfan syndrome, Ehlers-Danlos syndrome, homocystinuria, Hunter-Hurler syndrome, and mitral valve prolapse.

This condition can result in palpitations, tachycardia, dyspnea, and impaired cardiac function. However, the heart and great vessels are rarely compressed, and there may be no heart disease, despite the apparent (though misleading impression of) cardiac enlargement on the frontal chest radiograph.

Notes

Pectus Deformity Assoc: – Marfan
– Ehlers Danlos
– Homocystinuria
– MV Prolapse

→ Heart is displaced to Left

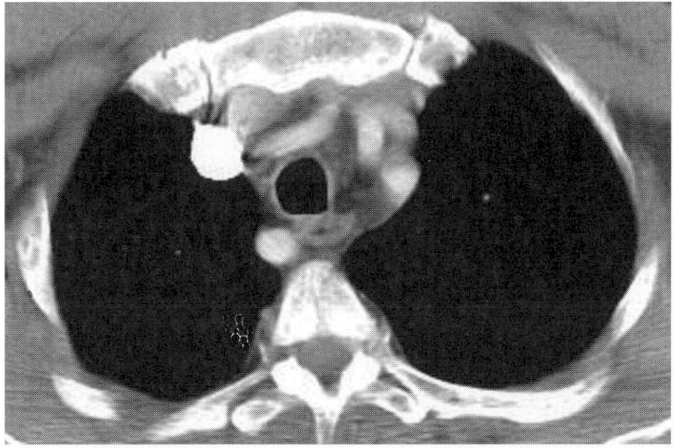

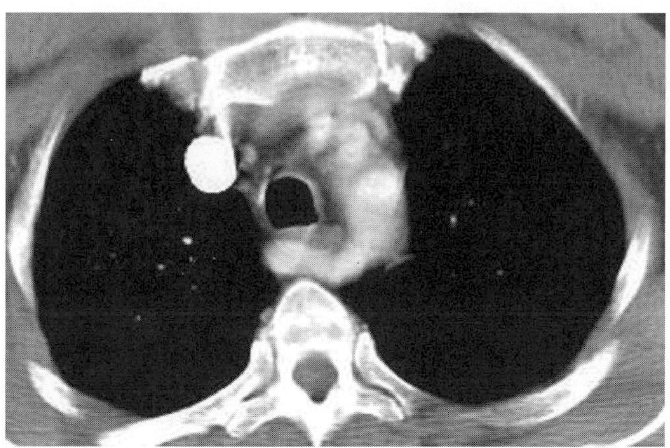

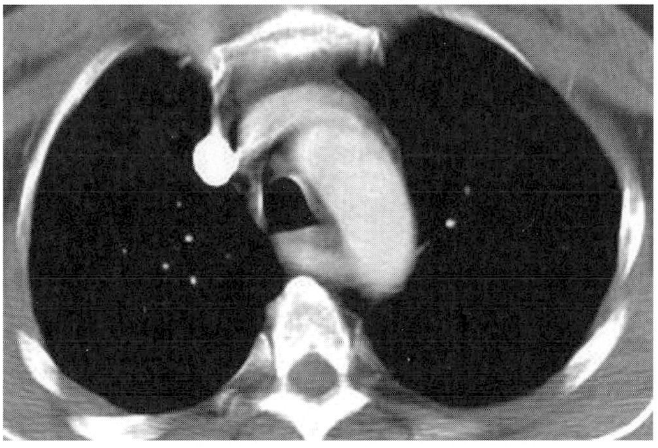

1. What is the arch anomaly shown?
2. Is this anomaly usually symptomatic?
3. Is this a vascular ring?
4. What is the incidence of this anomaly?

ANSWERS

CASE 13

Left Aortic Arch with Aberrant Right Subclavian Artery

1. Left aortic arch with aberrant right subclavian artery.
2. No.
3. No.
4. 0.5%

Reference

Harms J, Vogel T, Ennker J, Felix R, Hetzer R. Diagnostic evaluation and surgical management of the aberrant right subclavian artery. *Bildgebung* 61:299–303, 1994.

Cross-Reference

Cardiac Imaging: THE REQUISITES, 2nd edition, pp 406–407.

Comment

The CT scan demonstrates a left aortic arch. The right subclavian artery is aberrant, passing posterior to the esophagus.

A left arch with an aberrant right subclavian artery is a normal variant that occurs in 1/200 individuals. This anomaly is not a vascular ring, because the ligamentum arteriosum is on the left side and there is no structure completing the ring on the right. Because this lesion is not a vascular ring, there is no compression of the trachea and esophagus and symptoms are rare. The aberrant right subclavian artery may be dilated at its origin. This dilatation is known as a diverticulum of Kommerell. The course of the aberrant vessel is retroesophageal.

The anomaly can be identified incidentally on CT or with a barium swallow, which can demonstrate a slight posterior indentation of the esophagus.

Notes

(L) Arch c̄ Aberrant (R) subclavian

incidence - 1:200 (0.5%)

ring? - No

Sx's? - Not usually

Diverticulum of Kommerell = dilation of (R) subclavian @ its origin

CASE 14

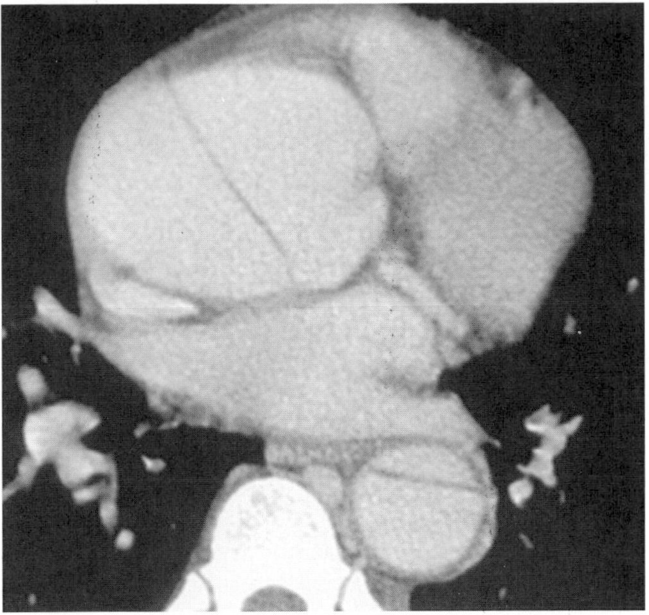

1. What is the diagnosis?
2. What is a Stanford type A dissection?
3. Name four life-threatening complications of this lesion.
4. How is this lesion treated?

CASE 15

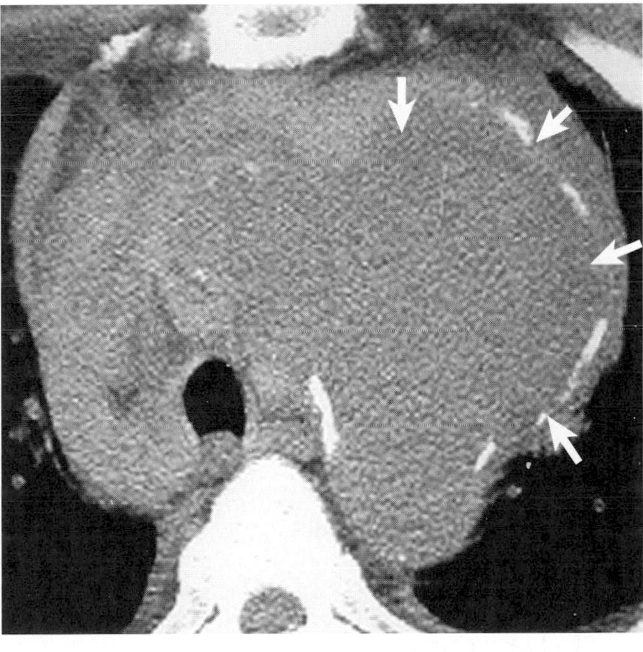

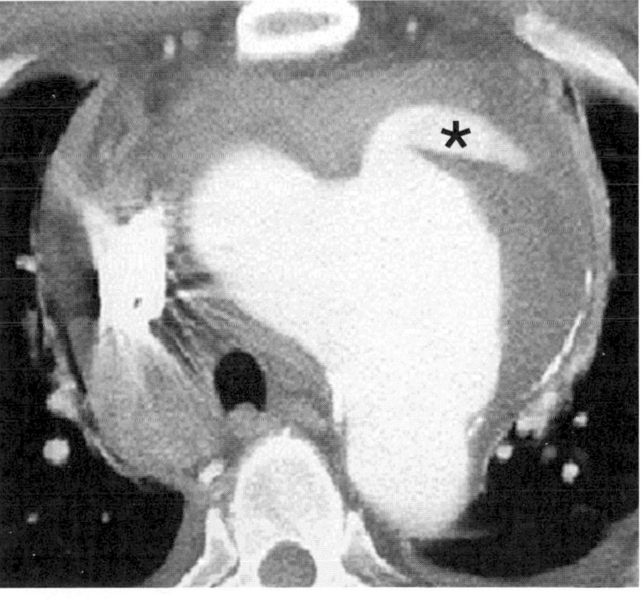

1. What is the source for the increased density in the mediastinum on the noncontrast CT scan?
2. What is represented by the asterisk (*) on the contrast-enhanced CT scan?
3. What is the diagnosis?
4. What threshold aortic diameter indicates high risk for this complication?

ANSWERS

CASE 14

Aortic Dissection—Stanford Type A

1. Aortic dissection, Stanford type A.
2. Dissection involving the ascending aorta, possibly extending into the descending aorta.
3. Dissection of the coronary arteries, dissection of the carotid arteries, pericardial hemorrhage and tamponade, and aortic valve rupture and acute aortic regurgitation.
4. With surgery.

Reference

Rubin GD. CT angiography of the thoracic aorta. *Semin Roentgenol* 38:115–134, 2003.

Cross-Reference

Cardiac Imaging: THE REQUISITES, 2nd edition, pp 371–380.

Comment

Aortic dissection is a separation of the aortic wall that results from intimal disruption. Typically blood flows in both the true and false lumina, although the false channel is sometimes thrombosed.

The most common predisposing factor for aortic dissection is hypertension. Other etiologies include annuloaortic ectasia (which is associated with connective tissue disorders such as Marfan syndrome or Ehlers-Danlos syndrome), bicuspid aortic valve, aortic aneurysm, and arteritis.

Aortic dissection can be classified as Stanford type A (involving the ascending aorta) or type B (involving the descending aorta only, distal to the left subclavian artery origin).

There are four major life-threatening complications of type A dissection: dissection of the coronary arteries resulting in myocardial infarction, dissection of the carotid arteries resulting in stroke, pericardial hemorrhage causing tamponade, and aortic valve rupture resulting in acute aortic regurgitation. Because of these potential complications, patients with type A dissection are usually treated surgically. In contrast, type B dissection usually can be managed medically, including the use of antihypertensive medication.

CT has high accuracy for the diagnosis of aortic dissection. MRI has similar accuracy and can serve as an alternative imaging modality, especially when CT is contraindicated or in the setting of a chronic dissection. Transesophageal echocardiography can be useful but may have lower specificity than CT or MRI.

Notes

Type A Complications (Life Threatening)
1) Coronary Artery Dissection ⇒ MI
2) Carotid Artery Dissection ⇒ CVA
3) Cardiac Tamponade 2° pericardial hemorrhage
4) Aortic Valve rupture ⇒ acute aortic regurg

CASE 15

Ruptured Aortic Aneurysm

1. Hematoma.
2. Penetrating ulcer.
3. Ruptured aortic arch aneurysm.
4. 6 cm.

Reference

Reddy GP, Higgins CB. MR imaging of the thoracic aorta. *Magn Reson Imaging Clin N Am* 8:1–15, 2000.

Cross-Reference

Cardiac Imaging: THE REQUISITES, 2nd edition, pp 398–401.

Comment

The noncontrast CT scan demonstrates a large saccular aneurysm of the aortic arch *(arrows)* and high-density material in the mediastinum, consistent with hematoma. The contrast-enhanced CT scan shows a large amount of atherosclerotic plaque within the aneurysm, as well as a penetrating ulcer (*). The findings are consistent with ruptured aortic aneurysm.

Aortic diameter diameter over 5 cm is called an aneurysm. The maximum diameter of the aorta is an important determinant of the risk of rupture. If the diameter is 6 cm or greater, the risk of rupture in the short term is greater than 30%.

Penetrating aortic ulcer occurs when atherosclerotic plaque ulcerates, disrupts the intima, and extends into the media. This can cause mural hemorrhage (intramural hematoma) and extension along the media, or occasionally aortic dissection or rupture.

CT findings of aneurysm rupture include high-density material in the aortic wall, pleural space, pericardium, or mediastinum. Indistinctness of the posterior aortic wall or close alignment of the posterior wall with the contour of the adjacent vertebral bodies is termed the "draped aorta" sign, which is suggestive of an early, contained rupture. On MRI, it is important to identify periaortic or mediastinal hematoma to make the diagnosis of aneurysm rupture. On spin-echo images, a hematoma appears as an area of high signal intensity, or sometimes intermediate signal intensity during the first few hours after bleeding.

Notes

CASE 16

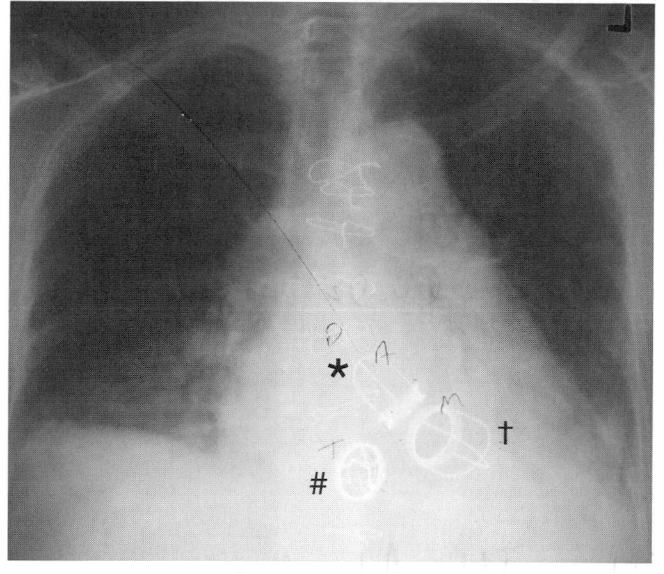

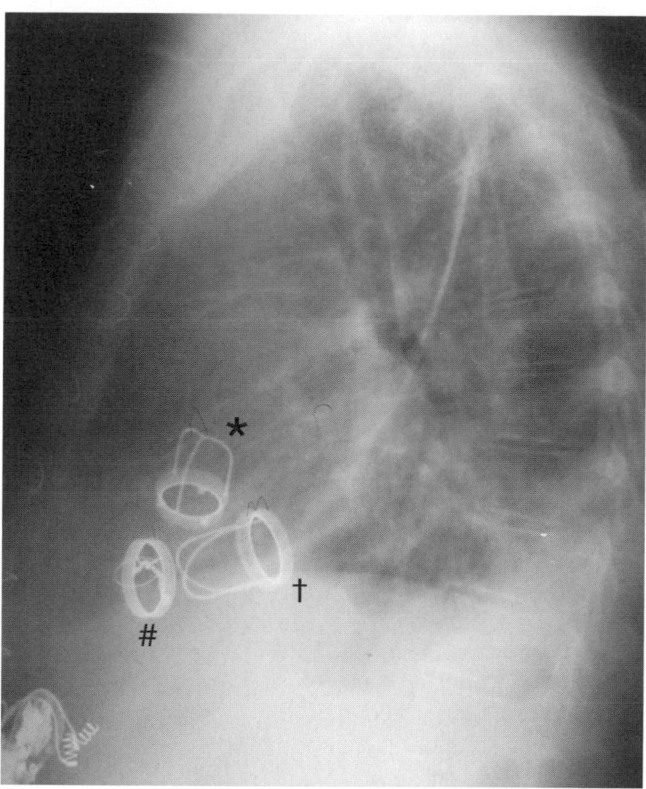

1. Which valve is indicated by the * symbol?
2. Which valve is indicated by the † symbol?
3. Which valve is indicated by the # symbol?
4. What is the most common cause of multivalve disease?

ANSWERS

CASE 16

Prosthetic Heart Valves

1. Aortic.
2. Mitral.
3. Tricuspid.
4. Rheumatic fever.

Reference

Steiner RM, Mintz G, Morse D, et al. The radiology of cardiac valve prostheses. *Radiographics* 8:277–298, 1988.

Cross-Reference

Cardiac Imaging: THE REQUISITES, 2nd edition, pp 64–66, 173–174, 184.

Comment

The chest radiographs demonstrate mechanical valves in the aortic, mitral, and tricuspid positions.

Rheumatic heart disease is the most common cause of three-valve disease. Patients with three-valve disease may present with heart failure and severe cardiomegaly. Surgery is complex with a mortality of approximately 5%. Typically, the prosthetic mitral and aortic valves are mechanical, and the tricuspid prosthesis may be mechanical or a bioprosthesis.

Mechanical prostheses have a variety of radiographic appearances, and some are even radiolucent. Patients who have a mechanical prosthesis require anticoagulation.

A bioprosthesis can be a heterograft (porcine), a homograft (from a cadaver), or an autograft, in which the patient's own pulmonary valve and root are used to replace the aortic valve and root; in this situation, a homograft is placed into the pulmonary position. Typically, bioprostheses have a single radiopaque ring.

Notes

CASE 17

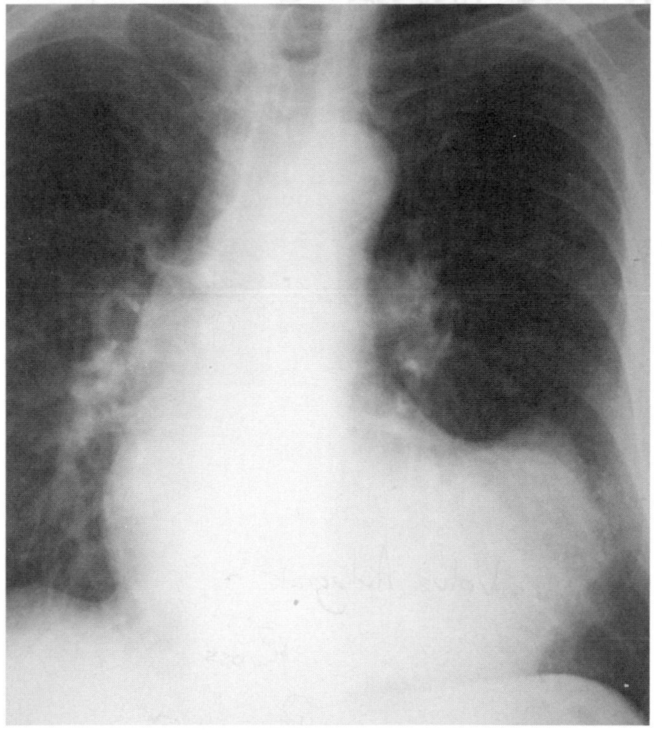

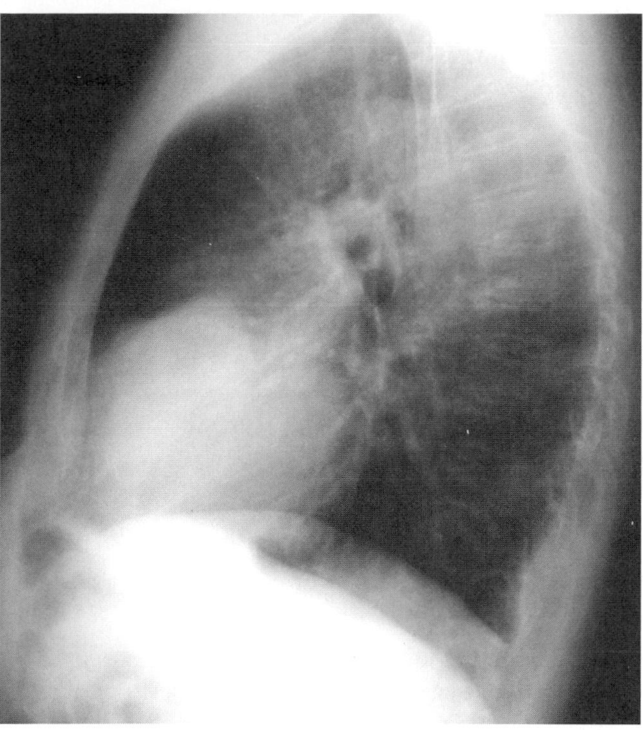

1. What is the most common cause of left ventricular aneurysm?
2. What is the typical location of a true left ventricular aneurysm?
3. What is the typical location of a false left ventricular aneurysm?
4. How can observation of the neck of the aneurysm on MRI or CT be used to differentiate a true aneurysm from a false aneurysm?

CASE 17

Left Ventricular True Aneurysm

1. Transmural myocardial infarction.
2. Anteroapical.
3. Inferoposterior.
4. If the neck is wide (greater than 50% of the aneurysm diameter), it suggests a true aneurysm. A narrow (less than 50%) neck suggests a false aneurysm.

Reference

White RD. MR and CT assessment for ischemic cardiac disease. *J Magn Reson Imaging* 19:659–675, 2004.

Cross-Reference

Cardiac Imaging: THE REQUISITES, 2nd edition, pp 234–241.

Comment

An anteroapical location of the aneurysm and a wide neck are consistent with a true aneurysm.

Left ventricular aneurysms result from a transmural myocardial infarction. True aneurysms have focal wall thinning and akinesis, with bulging during systole. Most true aneurysms are located in the anteroapical region of the left ventricle and have wide necks. A false aneurysm is actually a contained rupture. Most false aneurysms are inferoposterior in location and are connected to the left ventricle via a narrow neck.

With MRI or CT, true and false aneurysms can be differentiated on the basis of their necks.

Notes

CASE 18

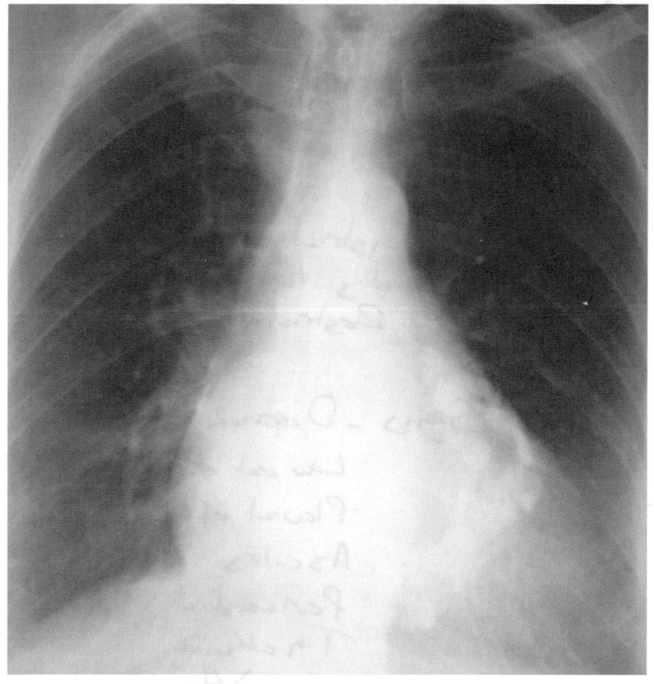

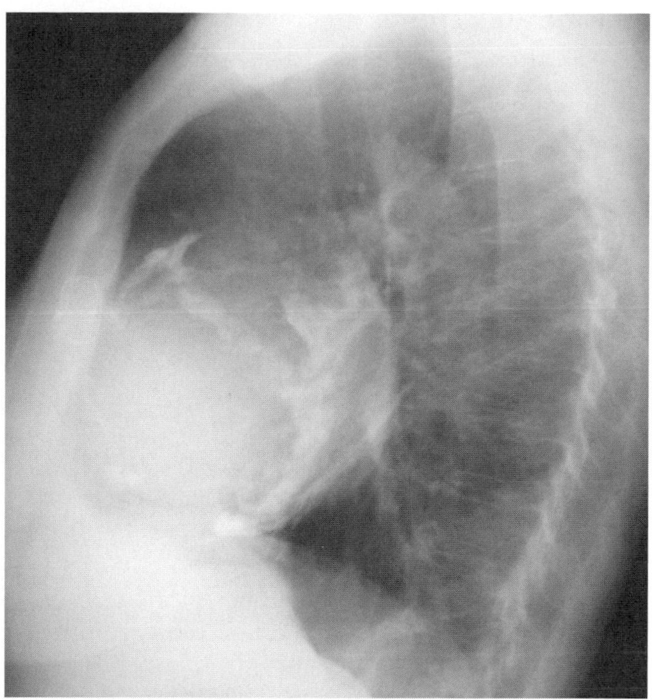

1. Which structure is calcified?
2. What is the diagnosis?
3. What is the most common cause of pericardial calcification?
4. What are the most commonly calcified areas of the pericardium?

CASE 18

Calcific Pericarditis

1. Pericardium.
2. Chronic calcific pericarditis.
3. Tuberculosis.
4. Atrioventricular and interventricular grooves, and the anterior and inferior heart borders.

Reference

Gowda RM, Boxt LM. Calcifications of the heart. *Radiol Clin North Am* 42:603–617, 2004.

Cross-Reference

Cardiac Imaging: THE REQUISITES, 2nd edition, pp 18, 253.

Comment

The chest radiographs demonstrate calcification of the pericardium. Pericardial calcification most often results from tuberculosis. Because tuberculous pericarditis is rare in industrialized countries, pericardial calcification occurs in less than 20% of patients with chronic pericarditis.

In chronic pericarditis, constrictive pericarditis can occur. Constrictive pericarditis is difficult to distinguish from restrictive cardiomyopathy. In the setting of constrictive/restrictive physiology, characterized by dyspnea, lower extremity edema, pleural effusions, and ascites, pericardial thickening of at least 4 mm (best seen on MRI or CT), pericardial calcification, or abnormal diastolic septal motion ("bounce") establish the diagnosis of constrictive pericarditis.

Notes

CASE 21

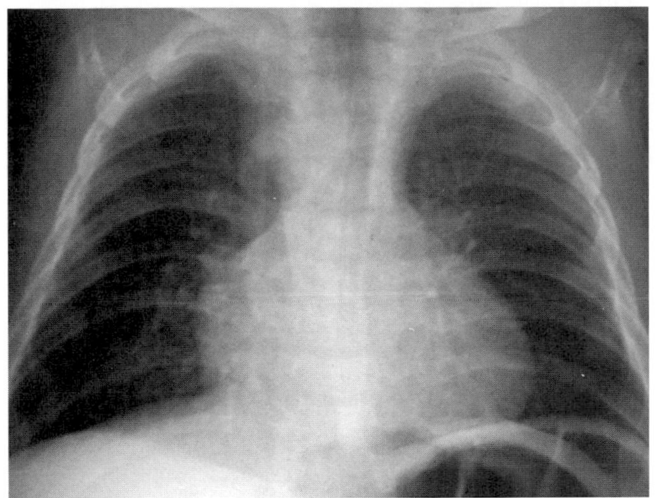

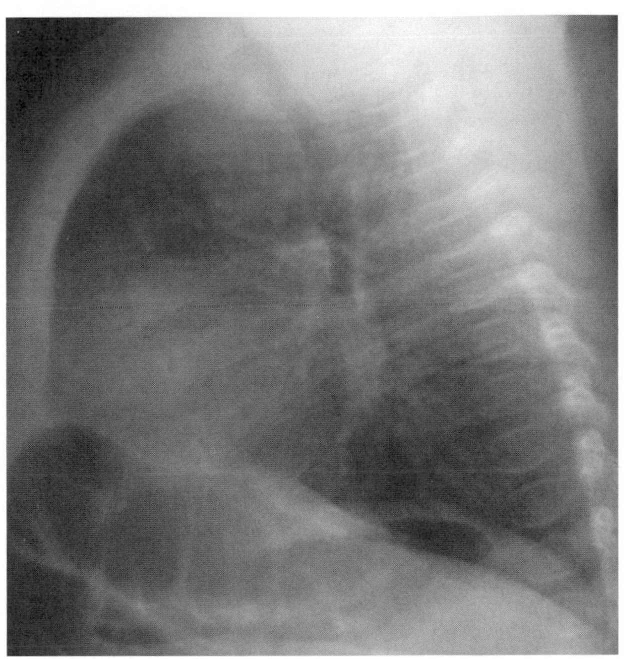

1. What are the four lesions that make up the tetralogy of Fallot?
2. Why are tetralogy of Fallot patients usually cyanotic?
3. What is the most common associated aortic arch anomaly?
4. How is pulmonary atresia with ventricular septal defect related to tetralogy of Fallot?

CASE 22

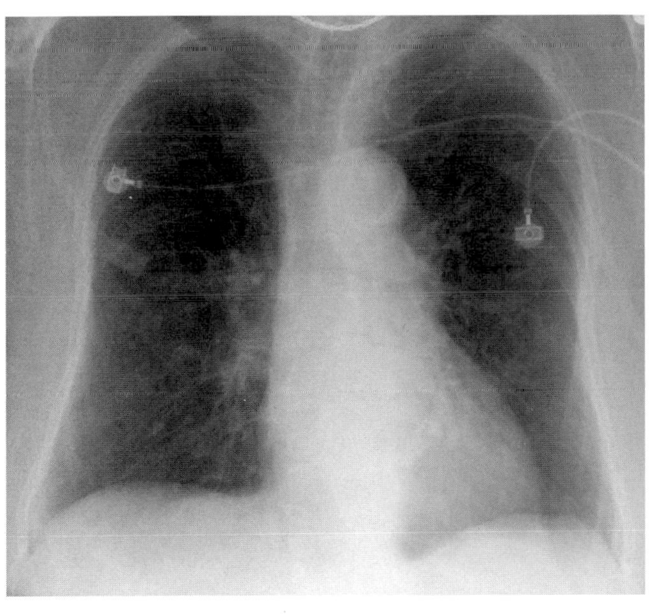

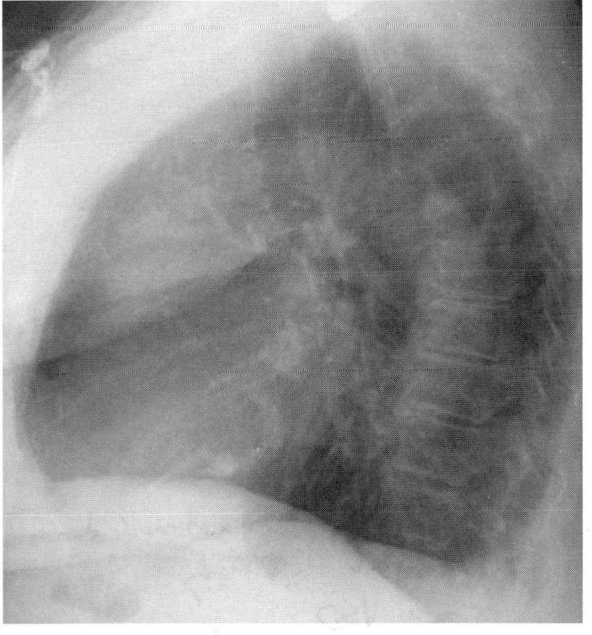

1. Which structure is calcified?
2. What letters of the alphabet can be used to describe the configuration of the calcification?
3. What is the associated valvular lesion?
4. What is the most common etiology of this calcification?

ANSWERS

CASE 21

Tetralogy of Fallot

1. Ventricular septal defect, overriding aorta, pulmonary infundibular stenosis, right ventricular hypertrophy.
2. Because the pulmonary outflow stenosis and ventricular septal defect result in a right-to-left shunt, deoxygenated blood is diverted away from the lungs and into the systemic circulation.
3. Mirror-image right aortic arch.
4. It is a severe variant of tetralogy.

Reference

Higgins CB. Radiography of congenital heart disease. In Webb WR, Higgins CB, editors: *Thoracic imaging: pulmonary and cardiovascular radiology*. Philadelphia, 2005, Lippincott Williams & Wilkins, pp 679–706.

Cross-Reference

Cardiac Imaging: THE REQUISITES, 2nd edition, pp 346–355.

Comment

The chest radiographs in an infant demonstrate normal-to-decreased pulmonary vascularity, normal size of the heart, and a right aortic arch. Angiography (not shown) demonstrated that it was a mirror-image right arch.

Tetralogy of Fallot is the most common cyanotic congenital heart disease in both children and adults. Most patients with tetralogy have decreased pulmonary vascularity, but vascularity can be normal if the infundibular stenosis is mild. Approximately 25% of patients have a right aortic arch. Pulmonary stenosis can occur at multiple levels, including subvalvular/infundibular (most common), valvular, supravalvular, and peripheral.

Pulmonary atresia with ventricular septal defect is a severe variant of tetralogy in which the pulmonary valve is atretic. Blood reaches the lungs via systemic-to-pulmonary collateral vessels.

In tetralogy, plain films typically demonstrate decreased vascularity, concavity of the pulmonary artery segment, and sometimes an upturned cardiac apex.

Notes

TOF (1) RV outflow track stenosis
(2) RV Hypertrophy
(3) VSD
(4) Overriding Aorta

CASE 22

Mitral Annular Calcification

1. Mitral annulus.
2. C, J, or O.
3. Mitral regurgitation.
4. Degeneration.

Reference

Gowda RM, Boxt LM. Calcifications of the heart. *Radiol Clin North Am* 42:603–617, 2004.

Cross-Reference

Cardiac Imaging: THE REQUISITES, 2nd edition, pp 15–16.

Comment

The plain films show calcification of the mitral annulus in a J shape. Other configurations include C and O shapes.

Mitral annular calcification is typically degenerative and related to aging. It occurs more frequently in women and in patients with chronic renal failure. When the calcification is extensive, it can lead to mitral regurgitation. It should be noted that calcification of the mitral valve leaflets themselves is associated with valvular stenosis, most commonly due to rheumatic disease.

Notes

Mitral Annular Calc ⇒ Degeneration
↳ Associated c̄ regurgitation
vs
Mitral Valve Calc ⇒ Rheumatic
↳ associated c̄ stenosis

CASE 23

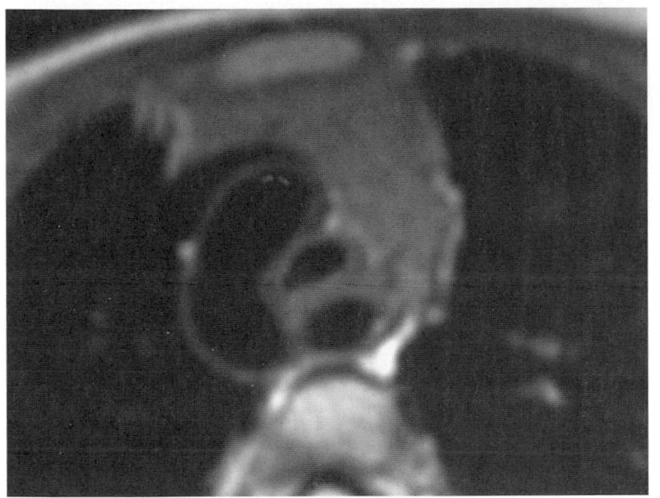

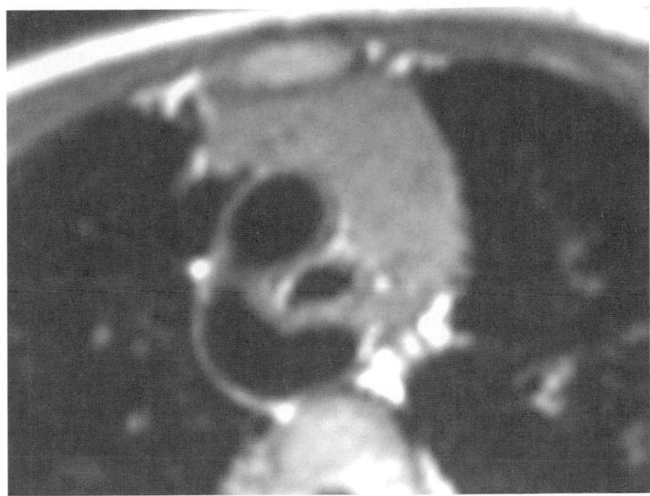

Axial spin-echo MR images.

1. What anomaly is shown?
2. Does the anomaly represent a vascular ring?
3. What are some common symptoms of this lesion?
4. Where does the anomalous vessel pass with respect to the esophagus?

CASE 24

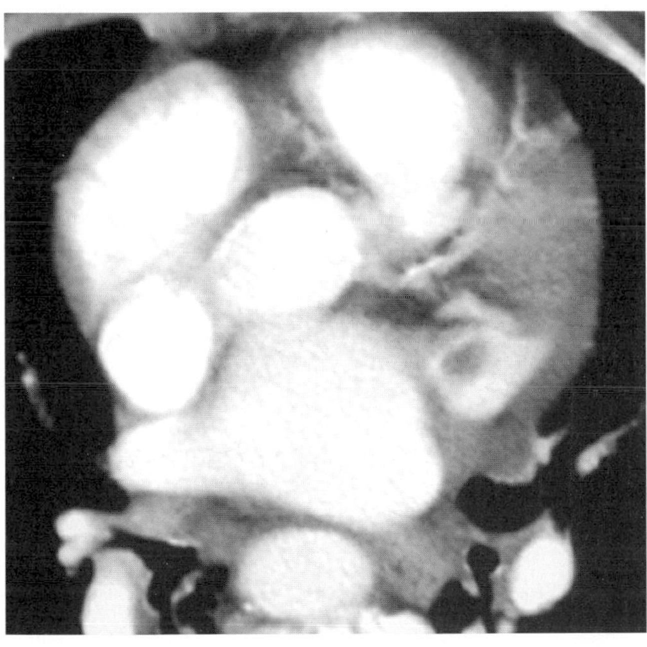

1. Where is the filling defect?
2. What is the most likely diagnosis?
3. What is the most likely etiology?
4. What are some complications of this lesion?

CASE 23

Right Aortic Arch with Aberrant Left Subclavian Artery

1. Right aortic arch with aberrant left subclavian artery.
2. Yes.
3. Wheezing, dyspnea, dysphagia.
4. Posterior to the esophagus.

Reference

Reddy GP, Higgins CB. Magnetic resonance imaging of congenital heart disease: evaluation of morphology and function. *Semin Roentgenol* 38:342–351, 2003.

Cross-Reference

Cardiac Imaging: THE REQUISITES, 2nd edition, p 407.

Comment

The MRI demonstrates a right aortic arch with a left subclavian artery that courses posterior to the esophagus. The trachea is substantially compressed.

A right aortic arch with an aberrant left subclavian artery is a vascular ring. The ring is completed by the left-sided ligamentum arteriosum. Because there is a ring around the trachea and esophagus, these two structures are compressed to a variable extent. The most common symptoms are wheezing, dyspnea, and dysphagia, and patients often exhibit these symptoms during early childhood. The retroesophageal aberrant left subclavian artery may have a dilated origin, known as a diverticulum of Kommerell, which tends to exacerbate the compression on the trachea and esophagus.

This type of right aortic arch is weakly associated (5% to 10%) with congenital heart disease, in contrast to the strong association of a mirror-image right arch (>95%).

MRI and CT can depict the vascular anatomy and the compression of the trachea and esophagus. Cine-MRI has the added advantage of demonstrating dynamic compression of the trachea during pulsation of the aorta and arch vessels.

Notes

CASE 24

Left Atrial Thrombus

1. Left atrial appendage.
2. Thrombus.
3. Atrial fibrillation.
4. Transient ischemic attack; stroke; infarct of kidney, spleen or bowel; peripheral embolization.

Reference

Tatli S, Lipton MJ. CT for intracardiac thrombi and tumors. *Int J Cardiovasc Imaging* 21:115–131, 2005.

Cross-Reference

Cardiac Imaging: THE REQUISITES, 2nd edition, p 75.

Comment

The contrast-enhanced CT scan demonstrates a nonenhancing mass (filling defect) in the left atrial appendage. Atrial fibrillation is the most common cause of left atrial thrombus.

Thrombus is the most common cardiac or paracardiac mass. Among cardiac and paracardiac neoplasms, secondary tumors occur at 40 times the rate of primary neoplasms. Secondary tumors can involve the heart by direct extension (most commonly lymphoma or lymphadenopathy metastatic from lung or breast carcinoma) or by hematogenous spread (most commonly lung or breast carcinoma, melanoma). Primary benign tumors of the heart include myxoma, lipoma, and rhabdomyoma (associated with tuberous sclerosis). Primary malignant neoplasms include angiosarcoma and rhabdomyosarcoma.

Thrombi in the left atrium can embolize, resulting in a transient ischemic attack; stroke; infarct of the kidneys, spleen, or bowel; or peripheral ischemia.

On CT scan, thrombi present as nonenhancing masses ("filling defects"). MRI is the most accurate imaging examination for differentiation of tumor from thrombus. Neoplasms enhance homogeneously or heterogeneously after administration of gadolinium-chelate contrast agent, whereas thrombi do not enhance. On gradient-echo (GRE) MRI, tumor usually shows intermediate signal intensity, and thrombus tends to demonstrate low signal intensity. Myxomas are often dark on GRE images.

Notes

CASE 25

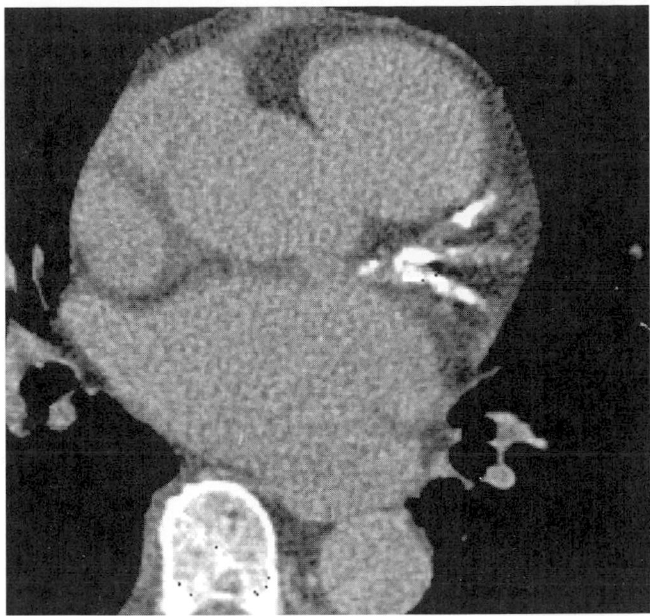

1. Where is the calcification?
2. What does the calcification indicate?
3. Does the calcification suggest that there is a stenosis at the site of calcification?
4. What type of CT scanner is required for coronary calcium assessement?

CASE 25

Coronary Artery Calcification

1. Coronary arteries.
2. Atherosclerosis.
3. No.
4. Electrocardiographically triggered electron-beam CT, or helical CT with electrocardiographic gating.

Reference

Ohnesorge BM, Hofmann LK, Flohr TG, Schoepf UJ. CT for imaging coronary artery disease: defining the paradigm for its application. *Int J Cardiovasc Imaging* 21:85–104, 2005.

Cross-Reference

Cardiac Imaging: THE REQUISITES, 2nd edition, pp 19–20.

Comment

The electron-beam CT image shows calcification of the left main, left anterior descending, left circumflex, and ramus medianus arteries.

Coronary calcification indicates atherosclerosis. CT can detect coronary calcification and has been used to identify patients with coronary artery disease. Frequently atherosclerosis builds up for decades before a patient develops symptomatic disease. Therefore, CT can be used to detect preclinical coronary artery disease. Although the quantity of coronary calcium corresponds to the total atherosclerotic burden, the site of calcification does not correlate directly with the location of stenosis.

Notes

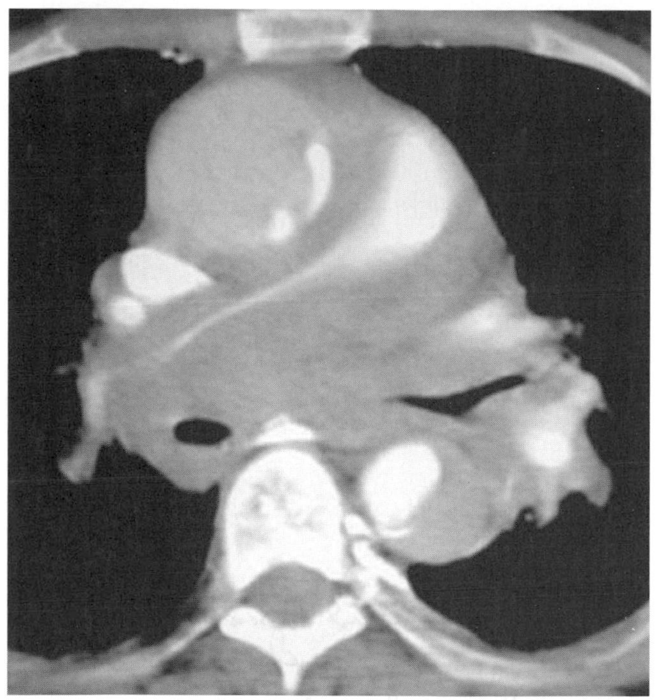

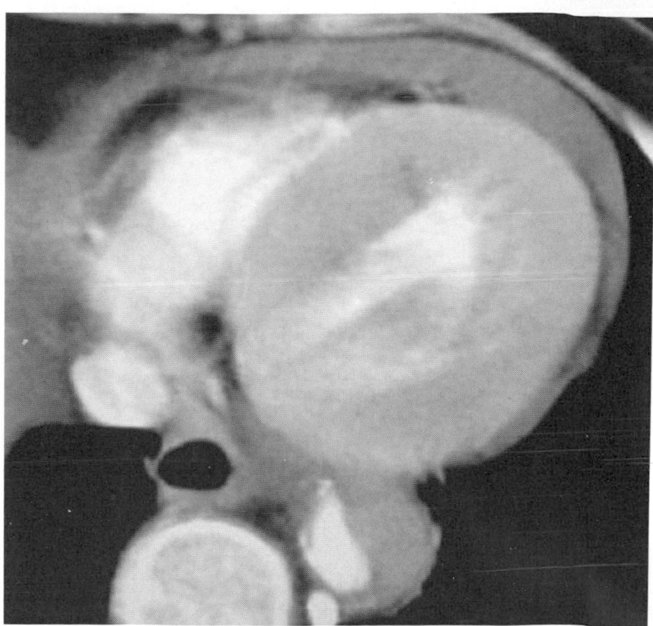

1. How would you classify this aortic dissection?
2. Is there an intramural hematoma?
3. What complication of dissection is present?
4. What is the utility of noncontrast CT for the evaluation of dissection?

CASE 26

Aortic Dissection—Stanford Type A with Pericardial Hemorrhage

1. Stanford type A or DeBakey type I.
2. No.
3. Pericardial hemorrhage.
4. Assessment of blood: intramural hematoma, thrombosed false lumen, pericardial hemorrhage. Assessment of displaced intimal calcification.

Reference

Rubin GD. CT angiography of the thoracic aorta. *Semin Roentgenol* 38:115–134, 2003.

Cross-Reference

Cardiac Imaging: THE REQUISITES, 2nd edition, pp 371–380.

Comment

The CT scan demonstrates a dissection involving the ascending and descending aorta. A dissection involving the ascending and descending aorta is classified as a type A dissection by the Stanford system or as a type I dissection by the DeBakey system. This CT demonstrates pericardial hemorrhage, which is one of the complications of a dissection that involves the ascending aorta.

Aortic dissection is a separation of the aortic wall that results from intimal disruption. Blood can enter the aortic wall through a tear in the intima, extending proximally and distally in the media, displacing the intima inward. Typically blood flows in both the true and false lumina, although the false channel is sometimes thrombosed.

The most common predisposing factor for aortic dissection is hypertension. Other etiologies include annuloaortic ectasia (which is associated with connective tissue disorders such as Marfan syndrome or Ehlers-Danlos syndrome), bicuspid aortic valve, aortic aneurysm, and arteritis.

Aortic dissection can be classified as Stanford type A (involving the ascending aorta) or type B (involving the descending aorta only, distal to the left subclavian artery origin). The DeBakey classification system identifies three types of dissection: type I involves the ascending aorta and extends into the descending aorta; type II involves the ascending aorta only; and type III involves the descending aorta only, beyond the origin of the left subclavian artery.

There are four major life-threatening complications of type A dissection: dissection of the coronary arteries resulting in myocardial infarction, dissection of the carotid arteries resulting in stroke, pericardial hemorrhage causing tamponade, and aortic valve rupture resulting in acute aortic regurgitation. Because of these potential complications, patients with type A dissection are usually treated surgically, with an ascending aortic graft. If the aortic valve is abnormal, the valve is replaced. In contrast, type B dissection usually can be managed medically, including the use of antihypertensive medications.

CT has high accuracy for the diagnosis of aortic dissection. MRI has similar accuracy and can serve as an alternative imaging modality, especially when CT is contraindicated or in the setting of a chronic dissection. Transesophageal echocardiography can be useful but may have lower specificity than CT or MRI.

Notes

Debakey I = Bad = ascending + descending
II = Ascending only
III = Descending only

A/I complications: - Dissection of the coronary artery ⇒ MI
- dissection of carotids ⇒ CVA
- Pericardial hemorrhage ⇒ Tamponade
- Aortic Valve rupture ⇒ Acute Aortic Regurg

CASE 27

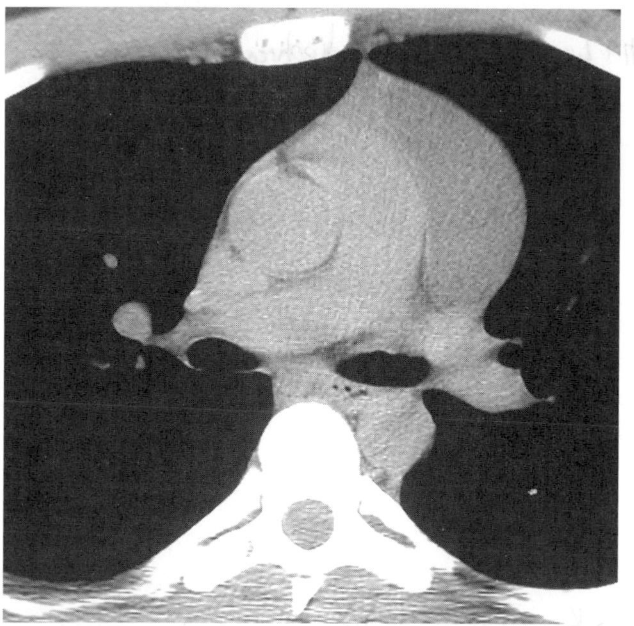

Noncontrast CT image.

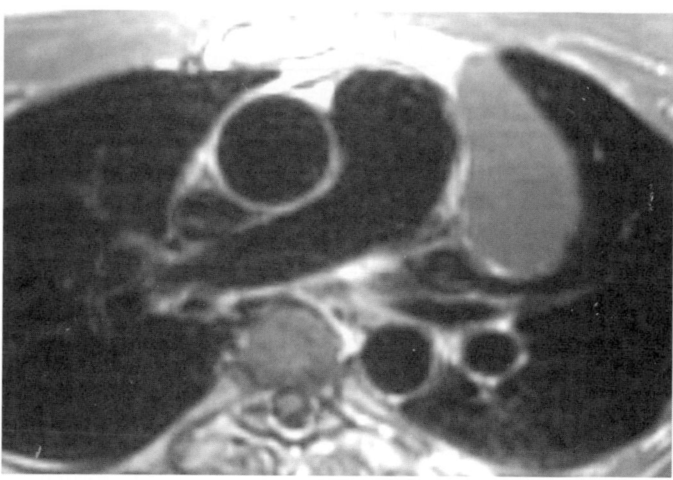

Axial spin-echo MR image.

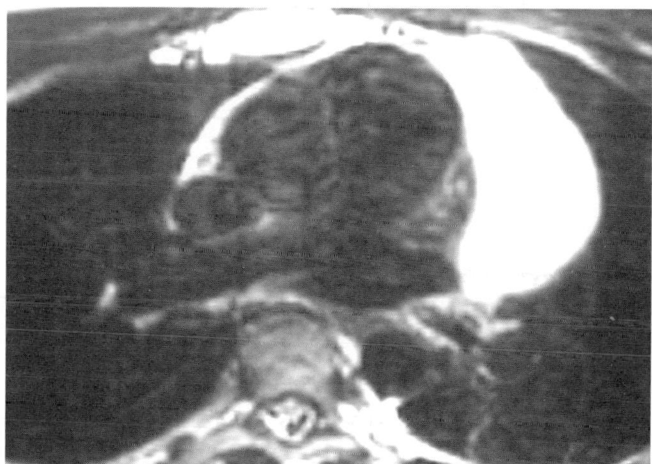

Axial T2-weighted MR image.

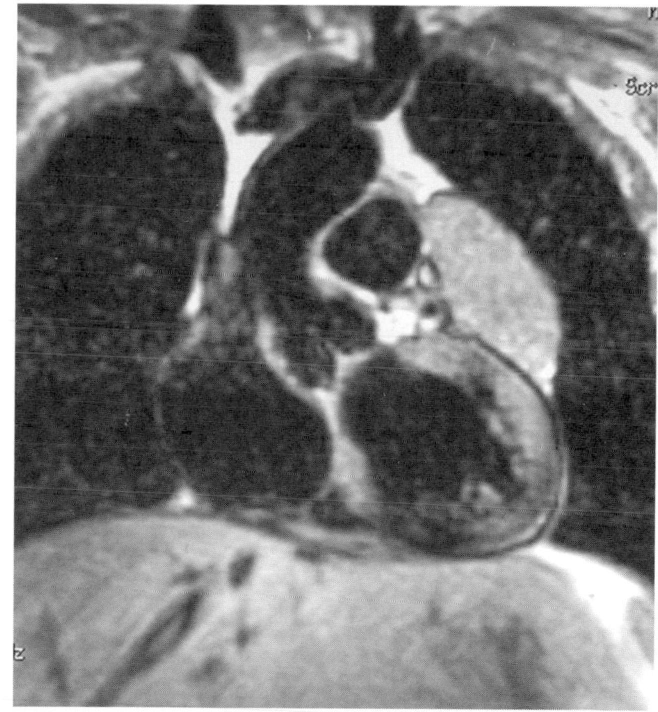

Coronal spin-echo MR image.

1. How is a pericardial cyst formed?
2. What is the most common location of a pericardial cyst?
3. What are the CT findings of a pericardial cyst?
4. What are the MR imaging findings of a pericardial cyst?

CASE 27

Pericardial Cyst

1. A portion of the embryonic pericardium is pinched off.
2. Right cardiophrenic sulcus.
3. Variable density (simple or complex fluid). Lack of enhancement when comparing noncontrast and postcontrast images.
4. Variable intensity—low (simple fluid), intermediate or high (complex fluid) on T1-weighted images. Lack of enhancement. High-signal intensity on T2-weighted images.

Reference

Wang ZJ, Reddy GP, Gotway MB, Yeh BM, Hetts SW, Higgins CB. CT and MR imaging of pericardial disease. *Radiographics* 23(Special Issue):S167–S180, 2003.

Cross-Reference

Cardiac Imaging: THE REQUISITES, 2nd edition, pp 256–258.

Comment

The CT scan demonstrates a well-circumscribed, homogeneous mass with the density of simple fluid. The T1-weighted MR image shows that the mass does not enhance. The T2-weighted MR image shows uniform high-signal intensity. These findings are diagnostic of a cyst. The location of this mass adjacent to the pericardium indicates that it is a pericardial cyst.

A pericardial cyst is a benign developmental lesion that is formed when a portion of the embryonic percardium is pinched off and isolated. It has a thin wall, contains clear fluid, and is well circumscribed. The two most common locations are the right and left cardiophrenic angles. When a pericardial cyst is located in another area of the mediastinum, it can be difficult to differentiate from a bronchogenic, esophageal duplication, neuroenteric, or thymic cyst.

On CT and MRI, pericardial cysts are round or ovoid and are contiguous with the normal pericardium. On MRI, these lesions typically exhibit signal characteristics consistent with that of simple cysts found elsewhere in the body. They present as low- to intermediate-signal masses on T1-weighted images, and high-signal intensity lesions on T2-weighted images. They do not enhance, unlike neoplasms.

Notes

Fair Game

CASE 28

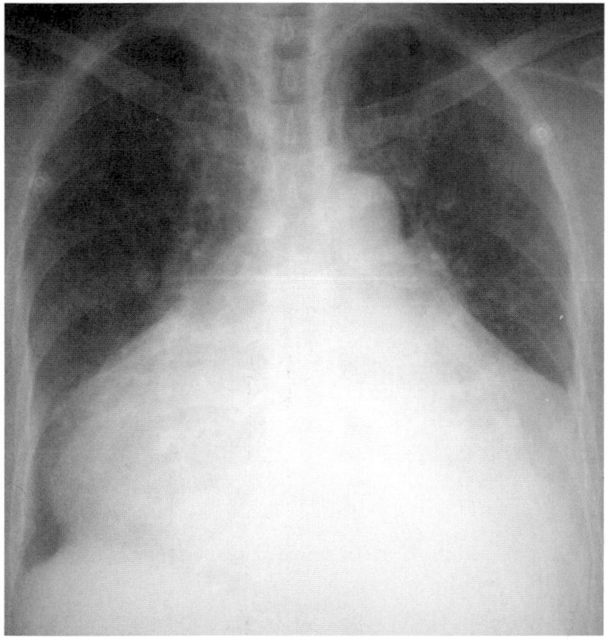

1. Which chambers are enlarged?
2. What is this appearance called?
3. What is the most likely diagnosis?
4. What is most common congenital cause of this lesion?

CASE 29

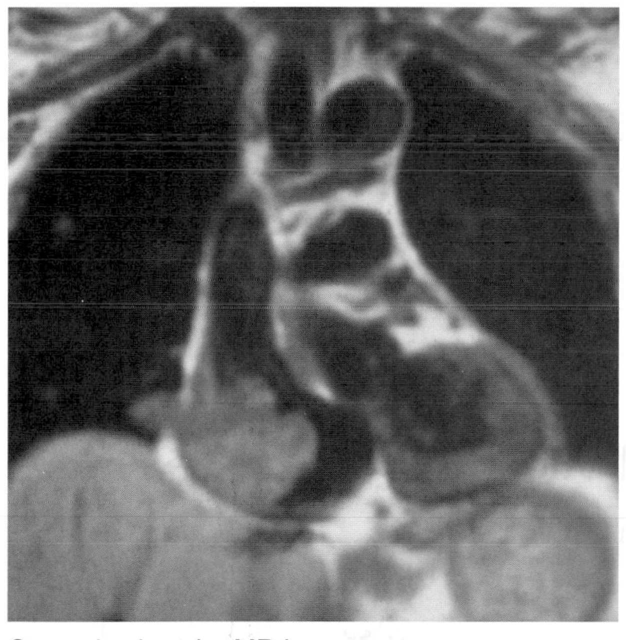

Coronal spin-echo MR image.

Axial spin-echo postgadolinium MR image.

1. Is the mass infiltrative?
2. Does the mass extend outside of the heart?
3. Is the mass benign or malignant?
4. If this is a primary tumor, what is the most likely diagnosis?

CASE 28

Tricuspid Regurgitation

1. Right atrium and ventricle.
2. "Wall-to-wall" heart.
3. Tricuspid regurgitation.
4. Ebstein anomaly.

Reference

Bonow RO, Cheitlin MD, Crawford MH, Douglas PS. Task Force 3: valvular heart disease. *J Am Coll Cardiol* 45:1334–1340, 2005.

Cross-Reference

Cardiac Imaging: THE REQUISITES, 2nd edition, pp 197–198.

Comment

The chest radiograph shows a massively enlarged cardiac silhouette. Differential diagnosis includes tricuspid regurgitation, dilated cardiomyopathy, and pericardial effusion.

Regurgitation can occur when there is an abnormality of one or more components of the tricuspid valve apparatus: the annulus, leaflets, chordae, papillary muscles, and right ventricular wall. Tricuspid regurgitation can be acquired or congenital. Acquired causes include pulmonary hypertension secondary to mitral valve disease (most common cause), papillary muscle rupture, rheumatic heart disease, bacterial endocarditis, and carcinoid syndrome. The most common congenital cause is Ebstein anomaly.

Chest radiographs demonstrate marked enlargement of the right atrium and ventricle. The heart can become massively enlarged, resulting in the so-called wall-to-wall heart. Echocardiography is used for further evaluation of regurgitation. Angiography and MRI can also be performed in selected cases.

When tricuspid regurgitation is secondary to mitral valve disease, treatment of the mitral disease can relieve the tricuspid regurgitation. In more severe cases, tricuspid valve replacement or annuloplasty is performed.

Notes

Wall to Wall heart DDx (3) – Pericardial effusion
– Tricuspid Regurgitation
– Dilated Cardiomyopathy

Tricuspid Regurg — Congenital ✱ Ebstein Anomaly
– Acquired – Pulm HTN 2° Mitral Valve Dz
• Rheumatic Heart Dz
– Bacterial endocarditis
– Carcinoid

CASE 29

Cardiac Angiosarcoma

1. Yes.
2. Yes.
3. Malignant.
4. Angiosarcoma.

Reference

Restrepo CS, Largoza A, Lemos DF, et al. CT and MR imaging findings of malignant cardiac tumors. *Curr Probl Diagn Radiol* 34:1–11, 2005.

Cross-Reference

Cardiac Imaging: THE REQUISITES, 2nd edition, p 266.

Comment

The MR image demonstrates a large, infiltrating mass involving the right atrium. The mass extends outside the heart (arrow). These findings indicate a malignant tumor. Definitive diagnosis is achieved by endomyocardial or open biopsy. This patient had an open biopsy, which yielded the diagnosis of angiosarcoma.

Approximately 98% of cardiac tumors are secondary tumors. The most common malignant primary cardiac tumor is angiosarcoma. Other primary malignant tumors are rare and include rhabdomyosarcoma, leiomyosarcoma, liposarcoma, and lymphoma.

MRI can be used to show tumor size and location, as well as cardiac function. Contrast-enhanced sequences can delineate tumor margins and invasion into adjacent structures. Note that the presence of enhancement does not signify malignancy—benign tumors enhance too! Features that suggest a primary malignant cardiac tumor include irregular or ill-defined margination, invasiveness, extension outside the heart, involvement of more than one chamber, central necrosis, large pericardial effusion, and lung nodules—which raise the possibility of metastases.

Notes

98% Cardiac Tumors = Mets (Secondary)

#1 Malignant Primary Tumor → Angiosarcoma

– also consider: – Rhabdomyosarcoma
– Leiomyosarcoma
– Liposarcoma

CASE 30

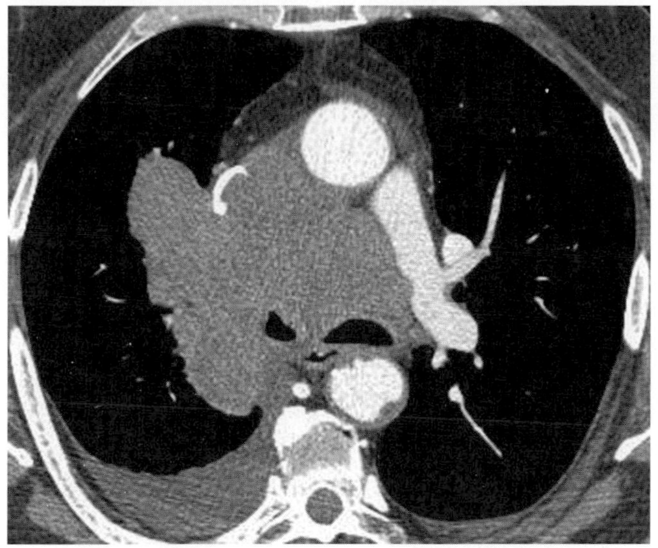

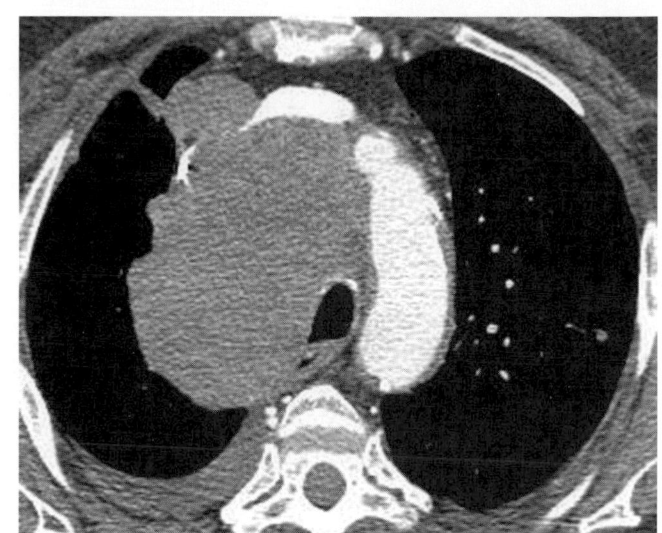

1. Which vessel is narrowed?
2. What is causing the narrowing?
3. What is the treatment in the acute setting?
4. Can this lesion be stented?

ANSWERS

CASE 30

Superior Vena Cava Syndrome

1. Superior vena cava.
2. Encasement by metastatic lung carcinoma.
3. Radiation therapy.
4. Yes, after radiation therapy relieves the acute symptoms.

References

Rowell NP, Gleeson FV. Steroids, radiotherapy, chemotherapy and stents for superior vena caval obstruction in carcinoma of the bronchus: a systematic review. *Clin Oncol (R Coll Radiol)* 14:338–351, 2002.

Remy J, Remy-Jardin M, Artaud D, Fribourg M. Multiplanar and three-dimensional reconstruction techniques in CT: impact on chest diseases. *Eur Radiol* 8:335–351, 1998.

Comment

The contrast-enhanced CT scan demonstrates metastatic mediastinal lymphadenopathy severely compressing the superior vena cava in a patient with bronchogenic carcinoma.

Signs and symptoms of superior vena cava syndrome are facial fullness and flushing, headache, upper extremity edema, and prominence of veins in the face and upper chest. The majority of cases are secondary to bronchogenic cancer. Other causes include histoplasmosis and tuberculosis involving the mediastinum, and caval thrombosis.

CT can be used to assess the mediastinum and to demonstrate the narrowing of the superior vena cava. MRI also can be performed to evaluate venous stenosis or occlusion and to identify the cause of narrowing.

Notes

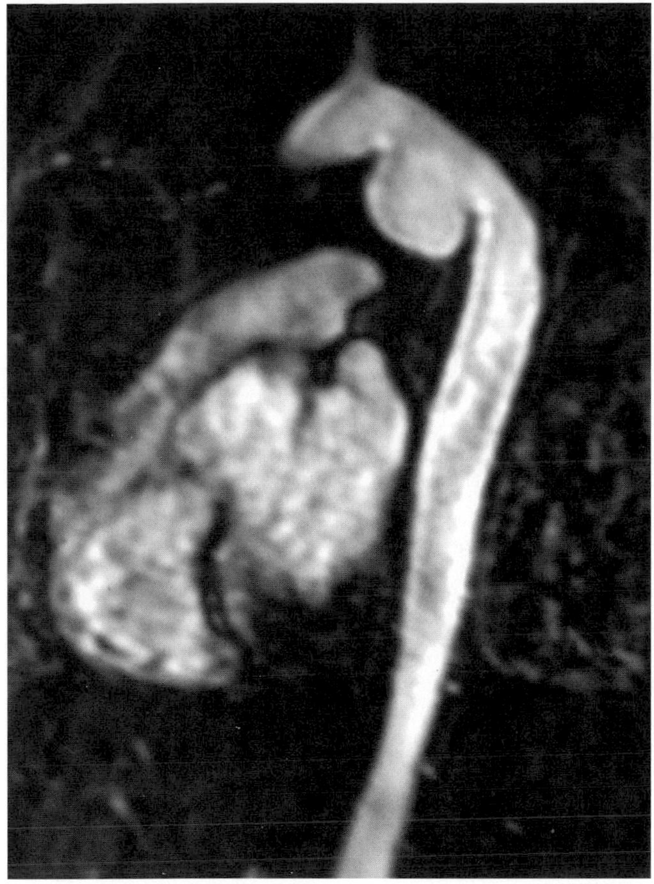

Gadolinium-enhanced MR angiogram.

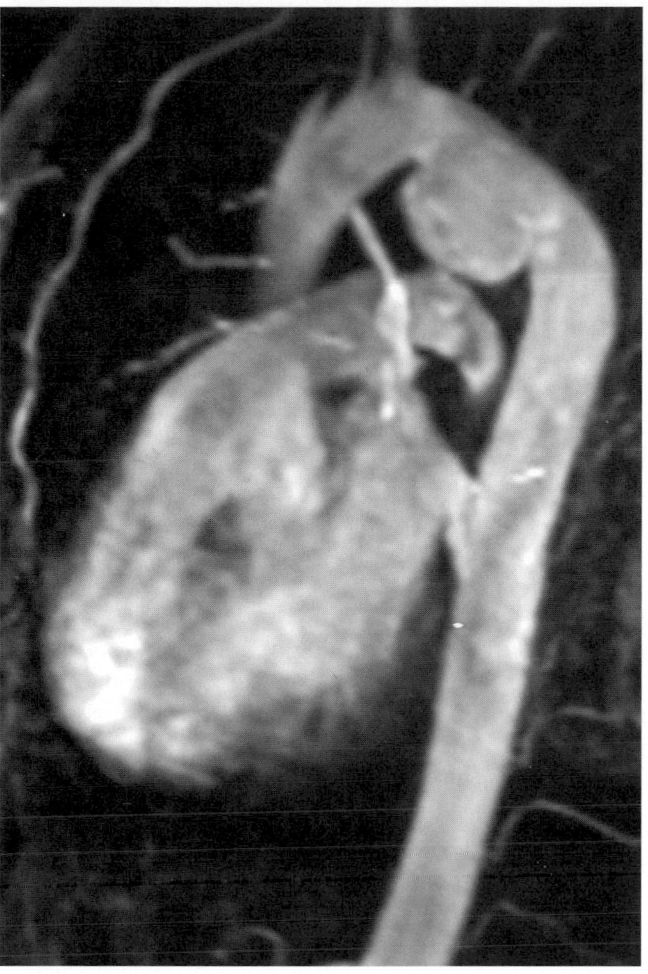

Maximum-intensity projection of gadolinium-enhanced MR angiogram.

1. The patient was involved in a motor vehicle collision several years before the MRI. What is the diagnosis?
2. What is the difference between a true aneurysm and a pseudoaneurysm of the aorta?
3. How can MRI differentiate a true aneurysm from a pseudoaneurysm?
4. How can this abnormality be treated?

ANSWERS

CASE 31

Traumatic Pseudoaneurysm of the Aorta—Chronic

1. Chronic pseudoaneurysm.
2. A true aneurysm is enlargement (diameter of 5 cm or greater) without disruption of the aortic wall. A pseudoaneurysm involves disruption of one or more layers of the wall.
3. A true aneurysm usually has a wide neck (at least 50% of the diameter of the aneurysm), and a pseudoaneurysm typically has a narrow neck.
4. Surgery or endovascular stent graft repair.

Reference

Gotway MB, Dawn SK. Thoracic aorta imaging with multislice CT. *Radiol Clin North Am* 41:521–543, 2003.

Cross-Reference

Cardiac Imaging: THE REQUISITES, 2nd edition, pp 395–397.

Comment

The MR image reveals an outpouching of the aorta with a narrow ostium. The location in the ductal region is characteristic of a traumatic pseudoaneurysm. Given that the patient was involved in a high-speed motor vehicle collision several years before the MRI, this image is consistent with a chronic pseudoaneurysm.

ATAI usually results from severe deceleration, injury due, for example, to a high-speed motor vehicle collision or a fall from a great height. The most frequent sites of injury are the isthmus (90%), the ascending aorta (5% to 10%), and the descending aorta near the hiatus (1% to 3%). Chronic pseudoaneurysm can develop in untreated long-term survivors.

A pseudoaneurysm is enlargement of the vessel associated with disruption of the wall. Causes of pseudoaneurysm include trauma, penetrating aortic ulcer, and infection (mycotic). On CT and MRI, a pseudoaneurysm is distinguished by a relatively narrow neck (<50% of the diameter of the aneurysm), as compared with the wide neck of a true aneurysm. Typically, pseudoaneurysms have a high risk of rupture, although the exact risk of rupture of a chronic traumatic pseudoaneurysm is not known. Because of the potential for catastrophic rupture, patients with a chronic traumatic pseudoaneurysm are usually advised to undergo open surgical repair or endovascular stent graft repair of the aorta.

Notes

CASE 32

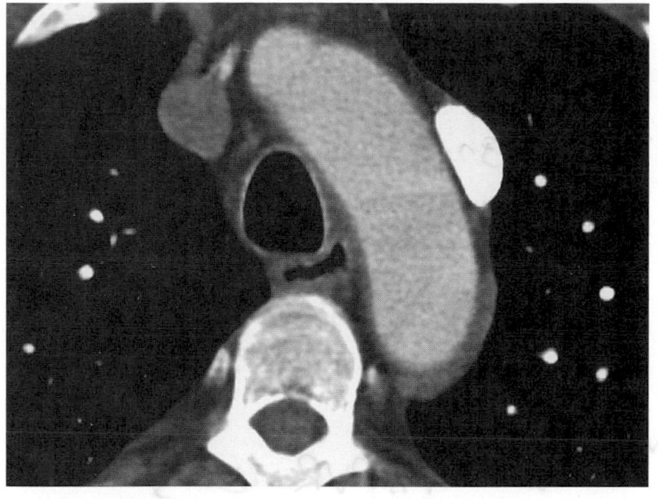

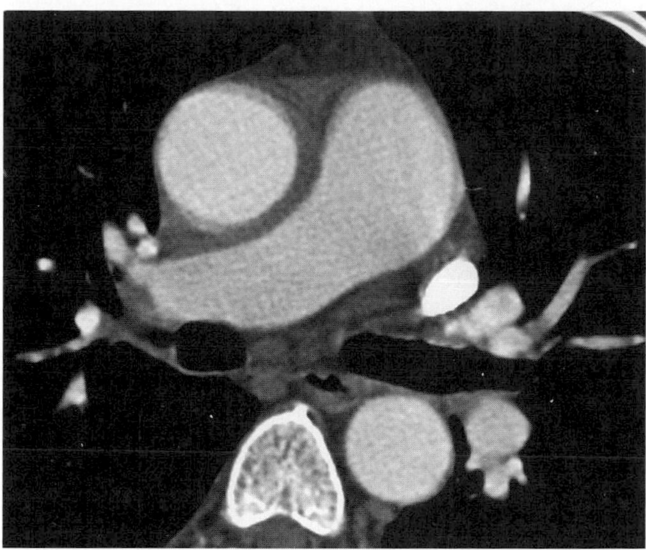

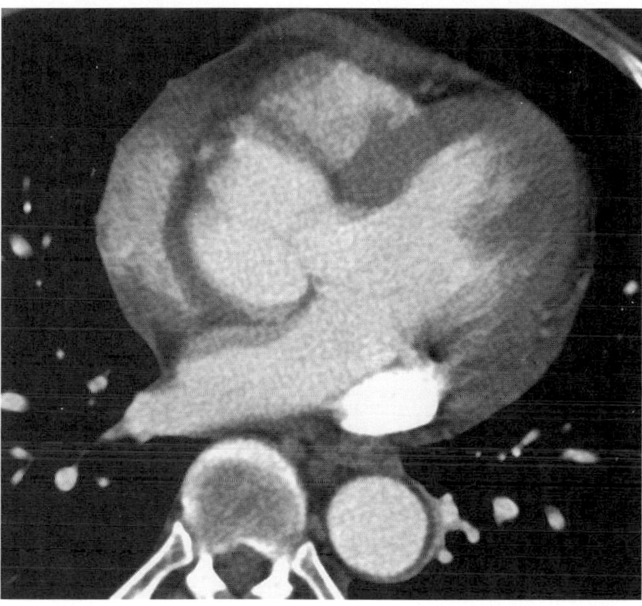

1. How can you distinguish a persistent left superior vena cava from a vertical vein related to partial anomalous pulmonary venous connection?
2. What is the most common site of drainage of a persistent left superior vena cava?
3. Is a right superior vena cava present in most patients with persistent left superior vena cava?
4. What is the name of the vessel that may connect the right and left superior venae cavae?

ANSWERS

CASE 32

Persistent Left Superior Vena Cava

1. Both structures derive from the fetal cardinal vein. Persistent left superior vena cava usually arises from the left brachiocephalic vein and drains into the coronary sinus. The vertical vein is related to partial anomalous pulmonary venous connection of the entire left lung or the left upper lobe. It arises in the hilum from the confluence of pulmonary veins and connects to the left brachiocephalic vein. It does not have an infrahilar component.
2. Coronary sinus.
3. Yes.
4. Bridging vein.

Reference

Minniti S, Visentini S, Procacci C. Congenital anomalies of the venae cavae: embryological origin, imaging features and report of three new variants. *Eur Radiol* 12:2040–2055, 2002.

Cross-Reference

Cardiac Imaging: THE REQUISITES, 2nd edition, pp 40–41.

Comment

The CT scan demonstrates a persistent left superior vena cava arising from the left brachiocephalic vein and draining into the coronary sinus.

Persistent left superior vena cava results when the left anterior cardinal vein persists after birth. The left brachiocephalic vein drains into the left superior vena cava, which usually connects to the coronary sinus. The coronary sinus may be dilated from the increase in flow, especially if there is no right superior vena cava. Most individuals with a persistent left superior vena cava have a right superior vena cava as well, and their anatomy is otherwise normal. The anomaly may be seen incidentally on a CT scan, or it may come to light after placement of a central venous catheter, pulmonary artery catheter, or a pacemaker.

Rarely, the left superior vena cava drains into the left atrium. In this situation, multiple severe cardiac anomalies may coexist, such as common atrium, atrioventricular canal defect, single ventricle, asplenia, and polysplenia. Persistent left superior vena cava is also associated with atrial septal defect, tetralogy of Fallot, as well as partial and total anomalous pulmonary venous connection.

Notes

CASE 33

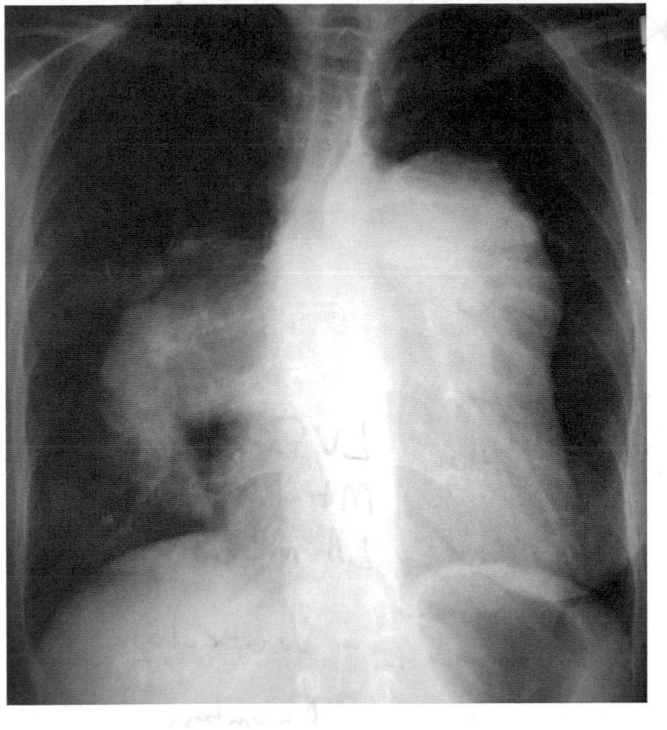

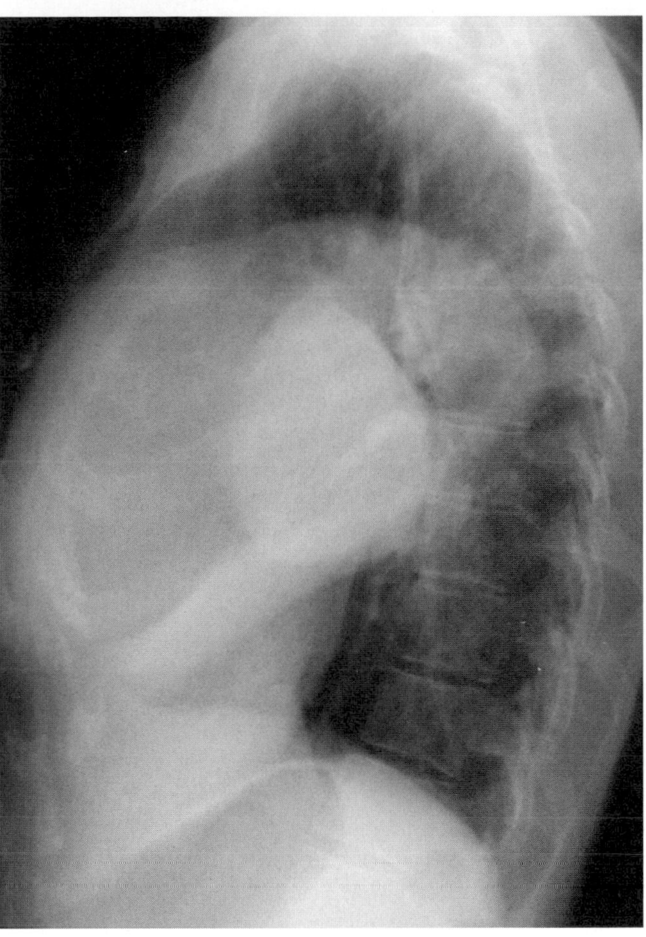

1. Is shunt vascularity present?
2. Does the patient have pulmonary hypertension?
3. This patient is acyanotic and has an intracardiac shunt. What is the most likely diagnosis?
4. If the pulmonary pressure exceeds systemic pressure, what syndrome can occur?

CASE 33

Eisenmenger Syndrome: Atrial Septal Defect

1. No.
2. Yes.
3. Atrial septal defect.
4. Eisenmenger syndrome: reversal of the shunt with right-to-left flow.

Reference

Wu JC, Child JS. Common congenital heart disorders in adults. *Curr Probl Cardiol* 29:641–700, 2004.

Cross-Reference

Cardiac Imaging: THE REQUISITES, 2nd edition, pp 324–326.

Comment

The chest radiograph shows marked enlargement of the central pulmonary arteries, consistent with pulmonary arterial hypertension.

When an atrial septal defect is longstanding, pulmonary pressure can increase dramatically and cause marked enlargement of the pulmonary arteries. Although there are a number of causes of pulmonary hypertension, it has been reported that an intracardiac shunt is the most common cause when there is massive pulmonary artery enlargement. As the pulmonary pressure rises, the left-to-right shunting decreases, and if the pulmonary pressure eventually exceeds systemic pressure, flow across the septal defect can reverse and become a right-to-left shunt. This is known as the Eisenmenger syndrome.

In the setting of Eisenmenger syndrome, the pulmonary vascularity is typically decreased. Patients may be cyanotic.

Notes

CASE 34

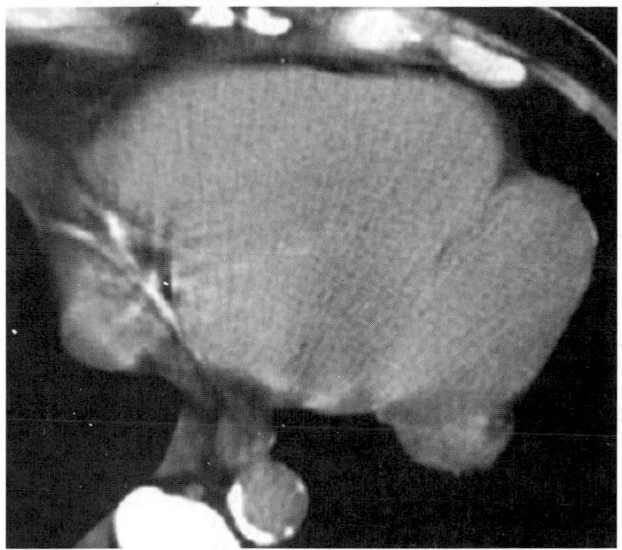

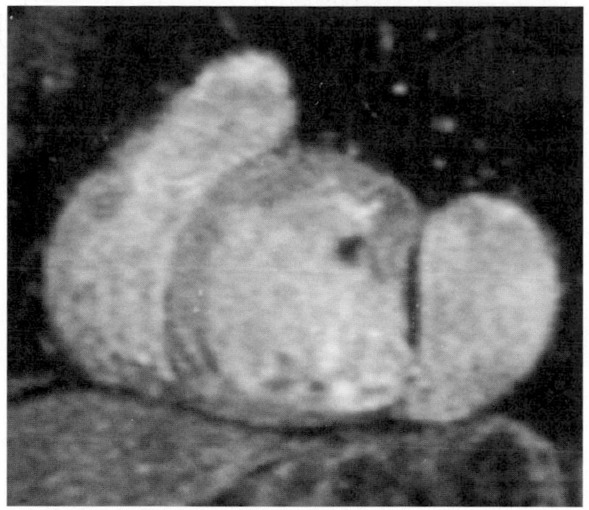

Coronal gradient echo cine-MR image.

1. Patient was referred for a CT-guided fine-needle aspiration of a mass in the chest. Would you perform a fine-needle aspiration of this lesion?
2. What is the diagnosis?
3. Can a false left ventricular aneurysm calcify?
4. How is a false aneurysm treated?

CASE 35

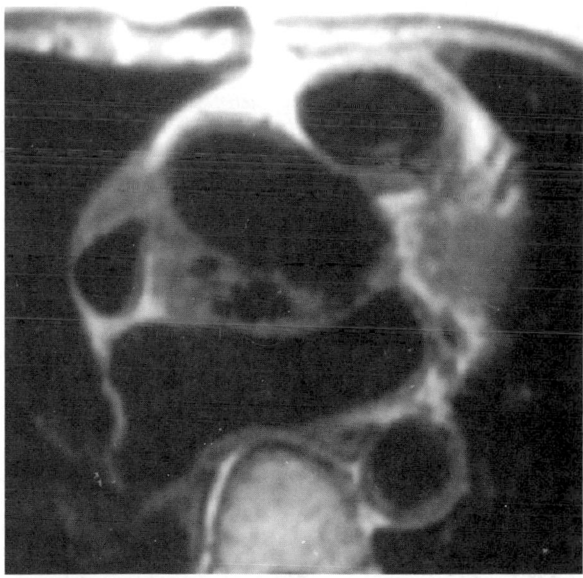

Axial spin-echo MR image.

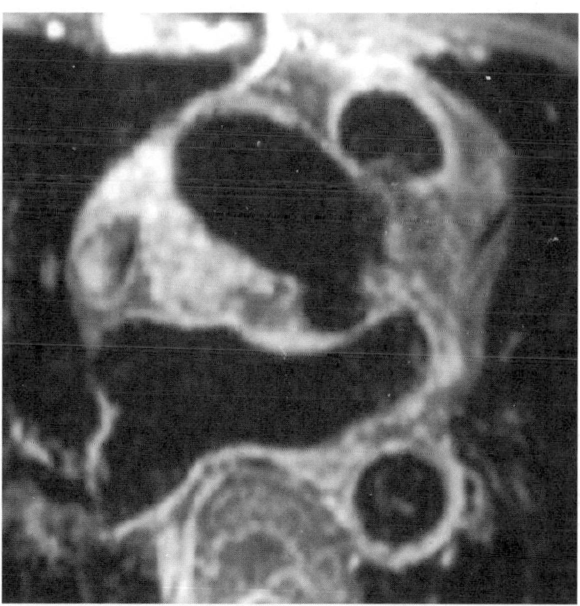

Axial spin-echo postgadolinium MR image with fat saturation.

1. This patient has infective endocarditis of her prosthetic aortic valve. What imaging modality is most commonly used for the diagnosis of endocarditis?
2. What is the enhancing area posterior to the aortic root?
3. What are the dark-signal areas posterior to the aortic root?
4. What are the most common pathogens that cause acute or subacute endocarditis?

ANSWERS

CASE 34

Left Ventricular False Aneurysm

1. No!
2. False aneurysm of the left ventricle.
3. Yes.
4. Because of the risk of rupture, false aneurysms are often surgically resected.

Reference

White RD. MR and CT assessment for ischemic cardiac disease. *J Magn Reson Imaging* 19:659–675, 2004.

Cross-Reference

Cardiac Imaging: THE REQUISITES, 2nd edition, pp 236–238.

Comment

The inferoposterior location of the aneurysm and the narrow neck (<50% of the diameter of the aneurysm) indicate a false aneurysm.

Left ventricular aneurysms result from a transmural myocardial infarction. True aneurysms have focal wall thinning and akinesis, with bulging during systole. Most true aneurysms are located in the anteroapical region of the left ventricle and have wide necks. A false aneurysm represents a contained rupture. Most false aneurysms are inferoposterior in location and are connected to the left ventricle via a narrow neck.

With MRI or CT, true and false aneurysms can be differentiated on the basis of their necks. Location is suggestive but not definitive for differentiating a true aneurysm from a false aneurysm. True aneurysms are usually managed medically unless there is substantial dysfunction such as heart failure, arrhythmia, or peripheral embolization of thrombus. False aneurysms, on the other hand, are usually resected because of the high risk of rupture.

Notes

True Aneurysms: Location: Anteroapical region
Neck: wide
Tx: Medical

False Aneurysm: Location: Inferoposterior
Neck: Narrow
Tx: Surgical

CASE 35

Periaortic Infection in Aortic Valve Infective Endocarditis

1. Echocardiography.
2. Periaortic infection.
3. Flow voids in a pseudoaneurysm. The larger dark-signal area is connected to the aortic root by a narrow neck.
4. *Streptococcus* and *Staphylococcus aureus.*

Reference

Reddy GP, Higgins CB. MR imaging of the thoracic aorta. *Magn Reson Imaging Clin N Am* 8:1–15, 2000.

Cross-Reference

Cardiac Imaging: THE REQUISITES, 2nd edition, pp 172, 268, 388–392.

Comment

The MR image demonstrates abnormal, enhancing soft tissue posterior to the aortic root, consistent with periaortic infection. Flow voids are seen as areas of low signal intensity. The larger flow void is connected to the aortic root by a narrow neck and is consistent with a pseudoaneurysm.

Infective endocarditis can be classified as acute or subacute. Acute bacterial endocarditis typically progresses in days to a severe systemic illness. Subacute endocarditis has a less toxic course and progresses over several weeks. *Streptococcus* and *Staphylococcus aureus* are the most common infective organisms. Predisposing factors include rheumatic disease, congenital heart disease, mitral valve prolapse, and intravenous drug use.

Although cine-MRI with steady-state free precession technique can be used for the identification of valvular vegetation to establish the diagnosis of endocarditis, echocardiography remains the imaging modality that is used most frequently for assessment of the cardiac valves.

Notes

Infective Endocarditis
risk factors: - Rheumatic Heart Dz
- Congenital heart Dz
- Mitral Valve prolapse
- IV Drug use

Organisms: - Streptococcus
- Staphylococcus

CASE 36

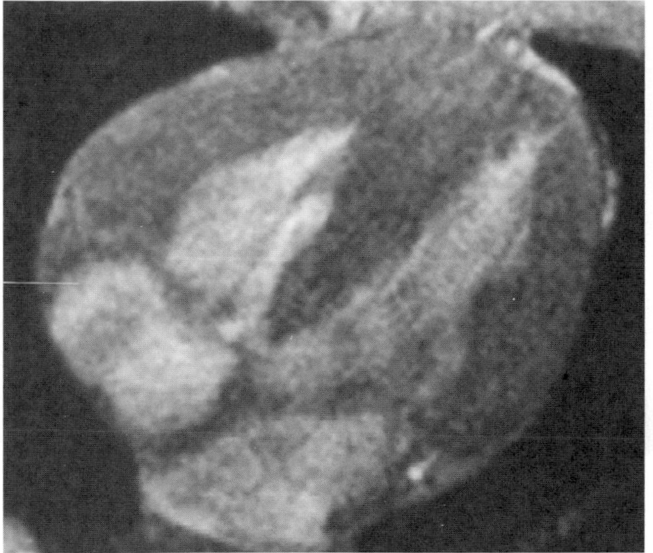

Horizontal long-axis gradient echo cine-MR image.

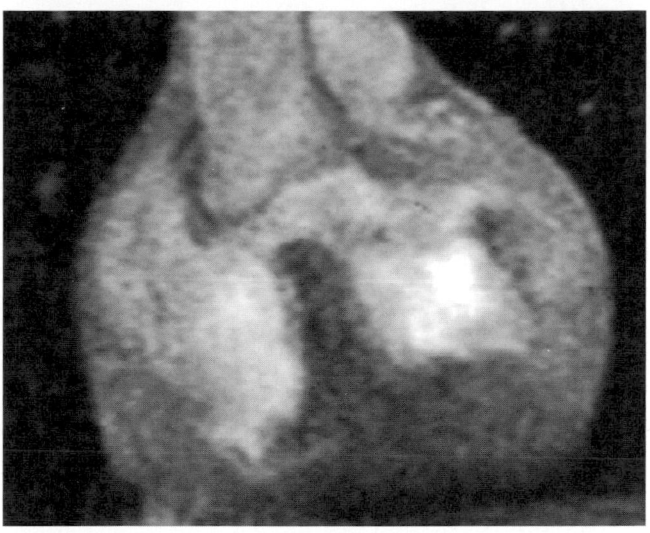

Coronal gradient echo cine-MR image.

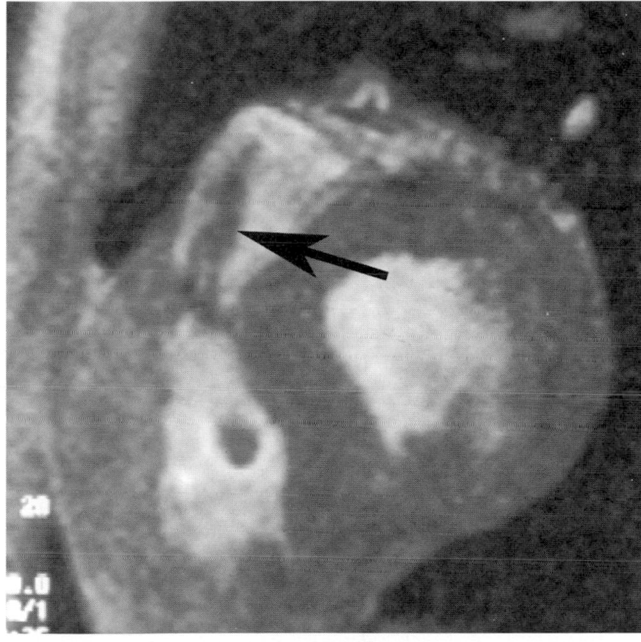

Sagittal gradient echo cine-MR image.
(Images courtesy of James Scatliff, MD.)

1. What is the diagnosis?
2. Is the RV wall normal?
3. What is an overriding aorta?
4. What does the low-signal line *(arrow)* represent?

ANSWERS

CASE 36

Tetralogy of Fallot on MRI

1. Tetralogy of Fallot.
2. No; it is hypertrophied.
3. An overriding aorta is positioned over the ventricular septal defect, allowing it to receive blood from both the right and left ventricles.
4. A poststenotic flow jet, indicating pulmonary outflow stenosis.

Reference

Reddy GP, Higgins CB. Magnetic resonance imaging of congenital heart disease: evaluation of morphology and function. *Semin Roentgenol* 38:342–351, 2003.

Cross-Reference

Cardiac Imaging: THE REQUISITES, 2nd edition, pp 346–355.

Comment

The cine-MR images show the four primary lesions of tetralogy of Fallot: an overriding aorta, a ventricular septal defect, pulmonary infundibular stenosis, and right ventricular hypertrophy.

Tetralogy of Fallot is the most common cyanotic congenital heart disease. Approximately 25% of patients with tetralogy have a right aortic arch, usually a mirror-image arch. Pulmonary stenosis can be present at multiple levels, including infundibular (most common), valvular, supravalvular, and peripheral.

MRI can be used for comprehensive evaluation of tetralogy of Fallot. Contrast-enhanced MR angiography can show the pulmonary artery sizes and can identify peripheral pulmonary arterial stenoses. Velocity-encoded cine–phase contrast images can be used to measure differential right and left pulmonary flow and to quantify regurgitation in the postoperative setting. Cine-MRI is employed for the quantitative appraisal of right ventricular function after surgery.

Notes

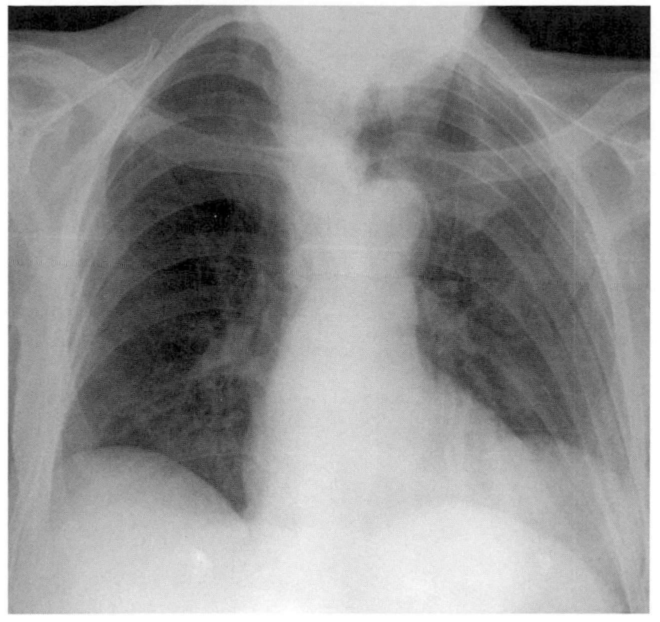

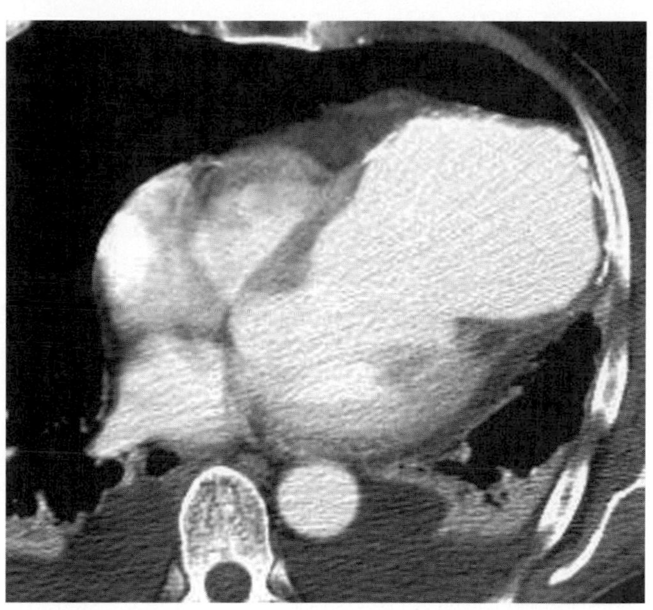

1. What is the diagnosis?
2. Is there thrombus within the mass?
3. Is there risk of peripheral embolization?
4. Should the mass be resected surgically?

CASE 37

Large Left Ventricular True Aneurysm

1. True aneurysm of the left ventricle.
2. Yes.
3. Yes.
4. Yes, if the aneurysm causes dysfunction such as heart failure, arrhythmia, or peripheral embolization.

Reference

White RD. MR and CT assessment for ischemic cardiac disease. *J Magn Reson Imaging* 19:659–675, 2004.

Cross-Reference

Cardiac Imaging: THE REQUISITES, 2nd edition, pp 234–241.

Comment

The plain film diagnosis is not obvious. On CT scan, the anteroapical location of the aneurysm and the wide neck are consistent with a true aneurysm. A small amount of thrombus is noted laterally.

Left ventricular aneurysms result from a transmural myocardial infarction. True aneurysms have focal wall thinning and akinesis, with bulging during systole. Most true aneurysms are located in the anteroapical region of the left ventricle and have wide necks. A false aneurysm represents a contained rupture. Most false aneurysms are inferoposterior in location and are connected to the left ventricle via a narrow neck.

With MRI or CT, true and false aneurysms can be differentiated on the basis of their necks. Differentiation is important because treatment is distinct for the two types of aneurysm. True aneurysms are usually managed medically unless there is substantial dysfunction such as heart failure, arrhythmia, or peripheral embolization of thrombus. False aneurysms, on the other hand, are usually resected because of the high risk of rupture.

Notes

True Aneurysm. Anteroapical

False Aneurysm. Inferoposterior

CASE 38

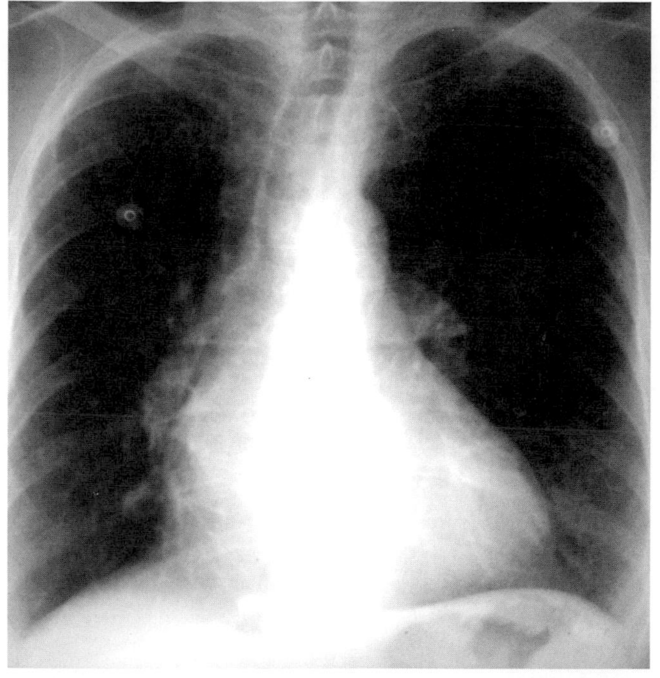

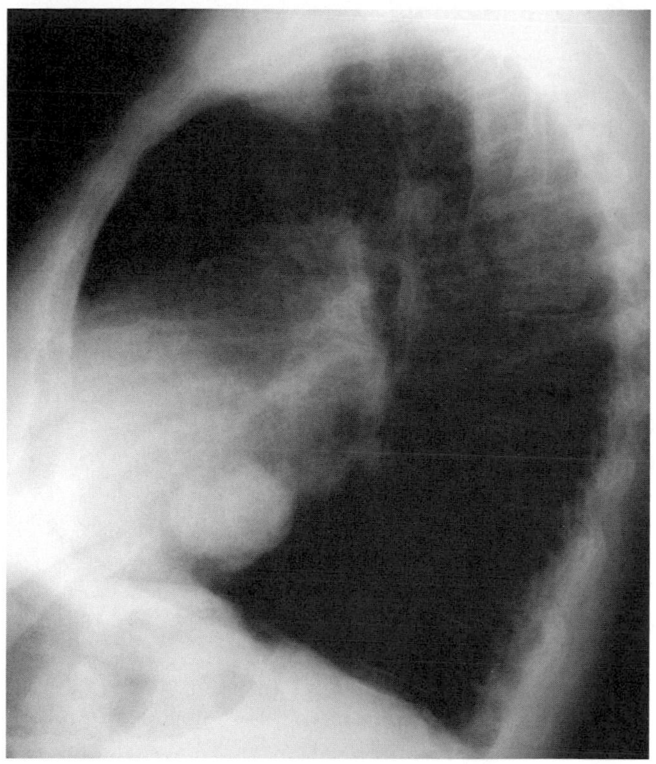

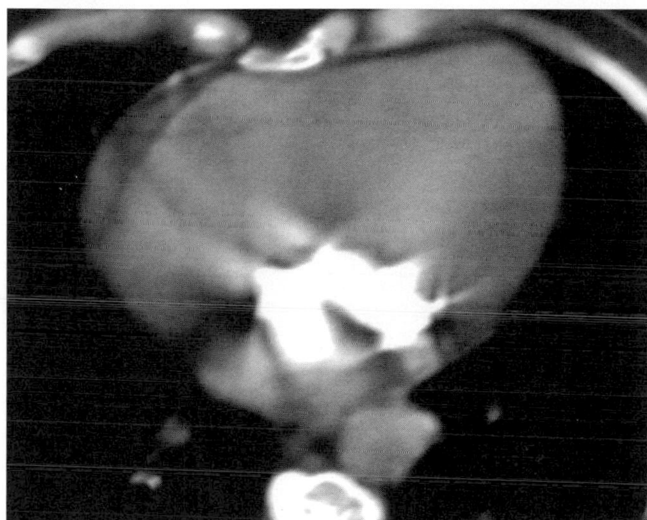

1. How many chambers are involved?
2. Does the mass extend outside the heart?
3. Is the mass benign or malignant?
4. What is the differential diagnosis?

CASE 38

Left Atrial Myxoma

1. One.
2. No.
3. Benign.
4. Calcified thrombus or myxoma.

Reference

Restrepo CS, Largoza A, Lemos DF, et al. CT and MR imaging findings of malignant cardiac tumors. *Curr Probl Diagn Radiol* 34:12–21, 2005.

Cross-Reference

Cardiac Imaging: THE REQUISITES, 2nd edition, pp 263–266.

Comment

Plain films demonstrate a mass projecting over the posterior aspect of the heart on the lateral view. The CT scan demonstrates a densely calcified, well-marginated mass in the left atrium. This is consistent with a benign mass. Differential diagnosis includes calcified thrombus and myxoma.

Myxoma is usually located in the left atrium and is one of the most common benign tumors of the heart. Patients with myxoma can be asymptomatic or develop symptoms of mitral stenosis or constitutional symptoms including fever, anemia, and elevated erythrocyte sedimentation rate. Myxomas can embolize to the systemic circulation and can cause transient ischemic attacks, stroke, or other systemic organ disease. Therefore, this tumor is usually resected even though it is benign.

This tumor is well-circumscribed and often has a narrow pedicle that is attached to the fossa ovalis of the atrial septum. A broad attachment to the atrial wall is less common. Myxomas can calcify, although dense calcification is uncommon, or become iron-stained. On spin-echo MRI, a myxoma typically appears as a mass of high signal intensity. Because of fibrosis, calcification, or iron deposition, myxomas can be dark on gradient-echo (GRE) MR images, mimicking the appearance of a thrombus. Therefore, it is important to look for contrast enhancement on spin-echo images, to differentiate myxoma from a thrombus, which does not enhance.

Notes

CASE 39

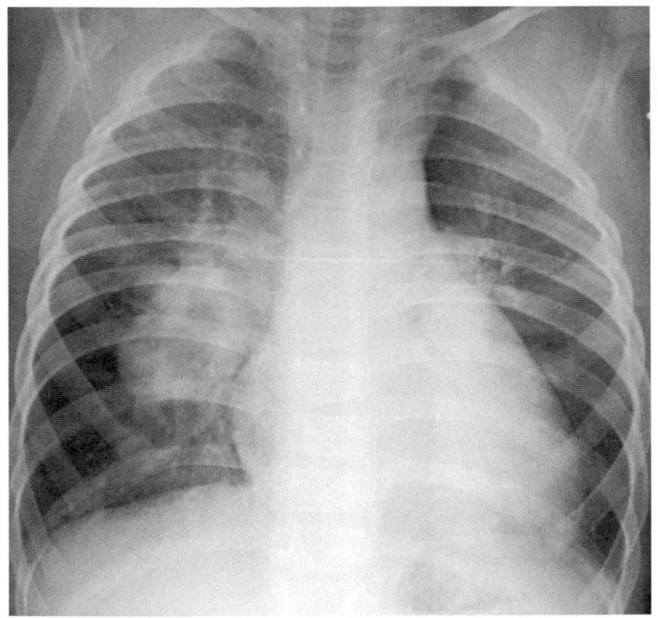

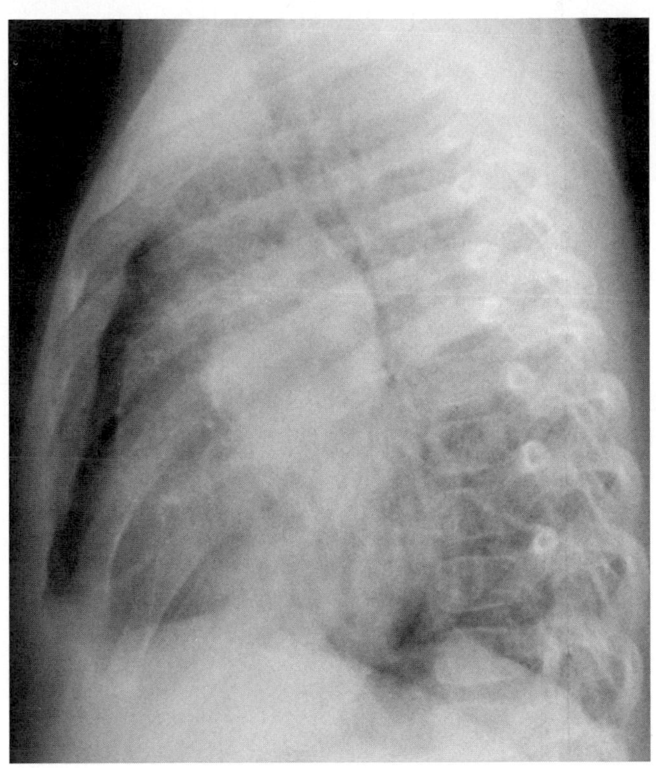

1. What vascular structures are enlarged?
2. What is the differential diagnosis?
3. This patient has tetralogy of Fallot. What is the most likely diagnosis?
4. Where is the primary obstructing lesion?

ANSWERS

CASE 39

Tetralogy of Fallot with Absent Pulmonary Valves

1. The central pulmonary arteries, especially the right pulmonary artery.
2. Pulmonary hypertension, pulmonary artery aneurysm, tetralogy of Fallot with absent pulmonary valves.
3. Tetralogy of Fallot with absent pulmonary valves.
4. Pulmonary valve.

Reference

Kirshbom PM, Kogon BE. Tetralogy of Fallot with absent pulmonary valve syndrome. *Semin Thorac Cardiovasc Surg Pediatr Card Surg Annu* 7:65–71, 2004.

Cross-Reference

Cardiac Imaging: THE REQUISITES, 2nd edition, p 193.

Comment

The chest radiographs demonstrate enlargement of the right pulmonary artery and (to a lesser extent) the left pulmonary artery. The main pulmonary artery enlargement is difficult to appreciate. This is an unusual appearance, given that in most patients who have tetralogy of Fallot with absent pulmonary valves, the main, left, and right pulmonary arteries are all markedly dilated. Frequently the lung volumes are large, a consequence of tracheobronchial compression.

Tetralogy of Fallot with absent pulmonary valves is characterized by a hypoplastic pulmonary annulus containing primitive valve tissue and aneurysmal dilation of the pulmonary arteries. The other lesions of tetralogy also exist in these patients. The marked pulmonary artery enlargement causes large airway compression, leading to early onset of respiratory distress.

Notes

DDx: Based on CXR

- Pulm HTN
- (R) PA aneurysm
- TOF c absent pulmonary valves

CASE 40

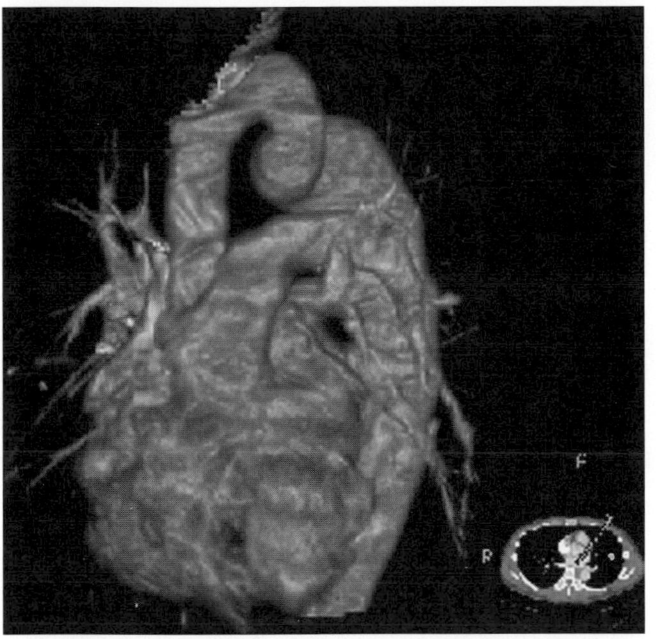

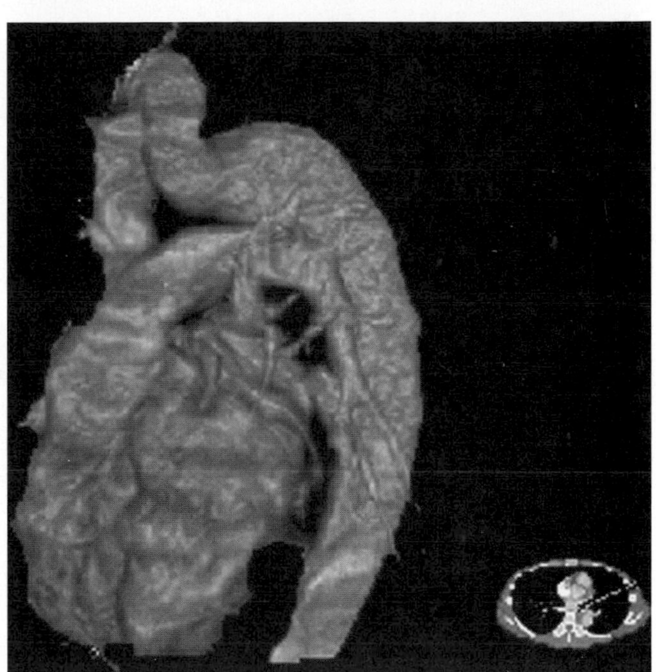

Volume-rendered reconstruction of CT. (Photo courtesy of Dr. Shangyun Ho, Chang-Hua, Taiwan.)

1. What is the diagnosis?
2. Why is the aorta kinked?
3. Docs collatcral flow develop in this condition?
4. Does rib notching occur?

ANSWERS

CASE 40

Pseudocoarctation of the Aorta

1. Pseudocoarctation.
2. The aorta is elongated and becomes kinked at the site of attachment to the ligamentum arteriosum.
3. No.
4. No.

Reference

Sebastia C, Quiroga S, Boye R, Perez-Lafuente M, Castella E, Alvarez-Castells A. Aortic stenosis: spectrum of diseases depicted at multisection CT. *Radiographics* 23(Special Issue):S79–S91, 2003.

Cross-Reference

Cardiac Imaging: THE REQUISITES, 2nd edition, p 420.

Comment

The CT scan demonstrates kinking of the aorta at the site of the ligamentum arteriosum. There is no significant narrowing of the lumen.

Pseudocoarctation is caused by elongation of the aortic arch and kinking at the site of attachment to the ligamentum arteriosum. The appearance of the aorta in pseudocoarctation is similar to that of true coarctation. However, there is no narrowing of the vessel lumen and no pressure gradient across the site of kinking. Therefore, collateral circulation does not develop and rib notching does not occur.

Notes

Pseudocoarctation caused by: elongation of the aortic arch + kinking @ ligamentum arteriosum attachment.

pressure gradient? No

No notching

No collaterals

CASE 41

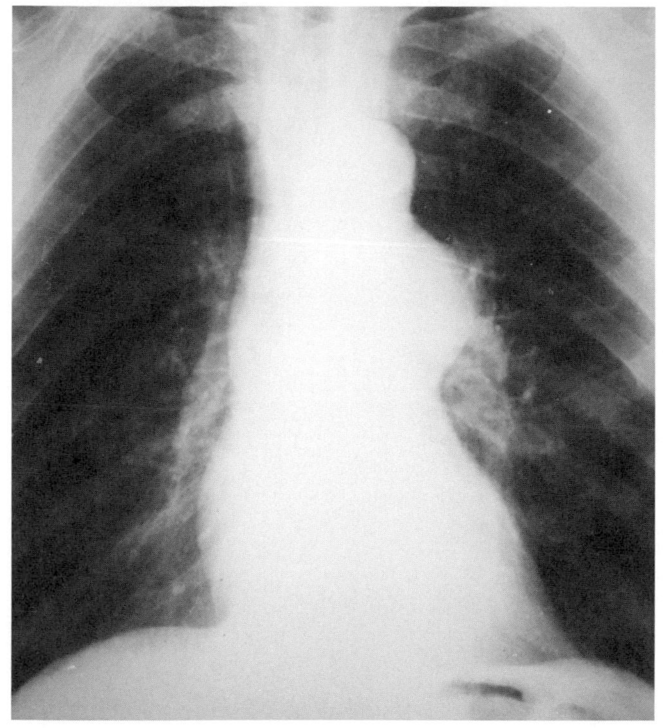

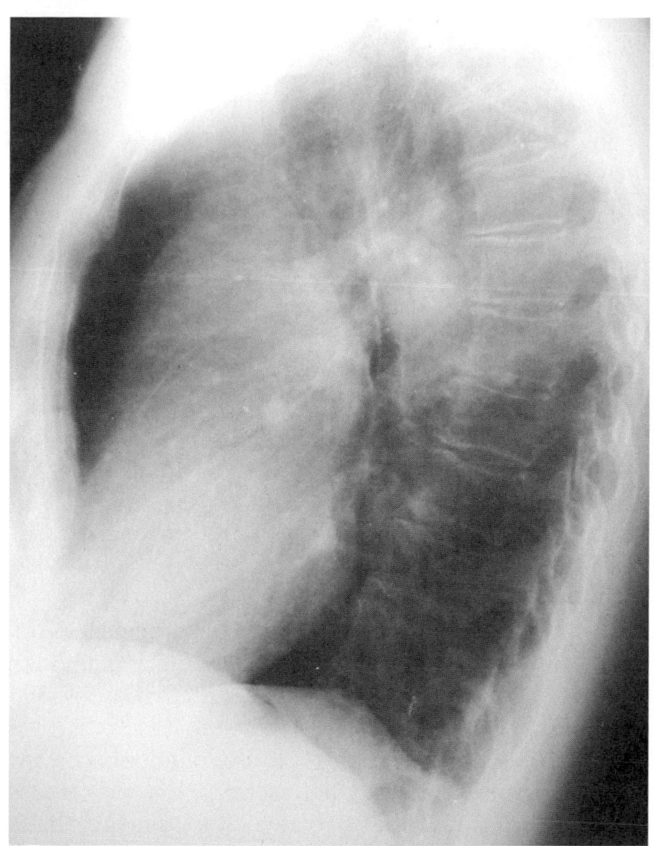

1. Which vascular structures are enlarged?
2. What is the most likely diagnosis?
3. What is the most common cause of this anomaly?
4. What is most common treatment in the neonatal period?

ANSWERS

CASE 41

Congenital Pulmonary Valve Stenosis

1. Main and left pulmonary arteries.
2. Congenital pulmonary valve stenosis.
3. Valve has a membrane with a central hole.
4. Balloon valvuloplasty.

Reference

Higgins CB. Valvular heart disease. In Webb WR, Higgins CB, editors: *Thoracic imaging: pulmonary and cardiovascular radiology*. Philadelphia, 2005, Lippincott Williams & Wilkins, pp 707–719.

Cross-Reference

Cardiac Imaging: THE REQUISITES, 2nd edition, pp 184–191.

Comment

The chest radiographs demonstrate enlargement of the main and left pulmonary arteries. The right pulmonary artery is normal. These findings are consistent with valvular pulmonary stenosis.

Pulmonary valve stenosis is most commonly congenital, resulting from a valvular membrane with a central hole, a bicuspid valve, or valve dysplasia (associated with Noonan syndrome).

Chest radiographic findings vary depending on patient age and associated abnormalities. In infants, a large thymus may obscure the central pulmonary arteries and the only sign of disease may be decreased pulmonary flow. In older children and adults, there is poststenotic dilatation of the main pulmonary artery and often of the left pulmonary artery. The right pulmonary artery is normal. Cardiac size is usually normal, unless the stenosis is severe enough to obstruct cardiac output.

Echocardiography demonstrates thickening and poor excursion of the valve leaflets and a jet across the lesion. Angiography demonstrates doming, thickening, and poor excursion of the valve leaflets. A jet of contrast agent can be seen passing across the valve.

Infants and young children can be treated with balloon valvuloplasty. One complication of balloon valvuloplasty is pulmonary regurgitation. Older children and adults usually require valve replacement.

Notes

CXR: enlarged main + (L) Pulm Arts
(R) Pulm Art nl

Pulm Valve Stenosis · DDx - Congenital
- valve membrane c̄ a hole
- bicuspid valve
- valve Dysplasia (Noonan Syndrome
- Pulm Stenosis
- ASD
- Hypertrophic Cardiomyopathy)

Tx: Balloon Valvuloplasty

CASE 42

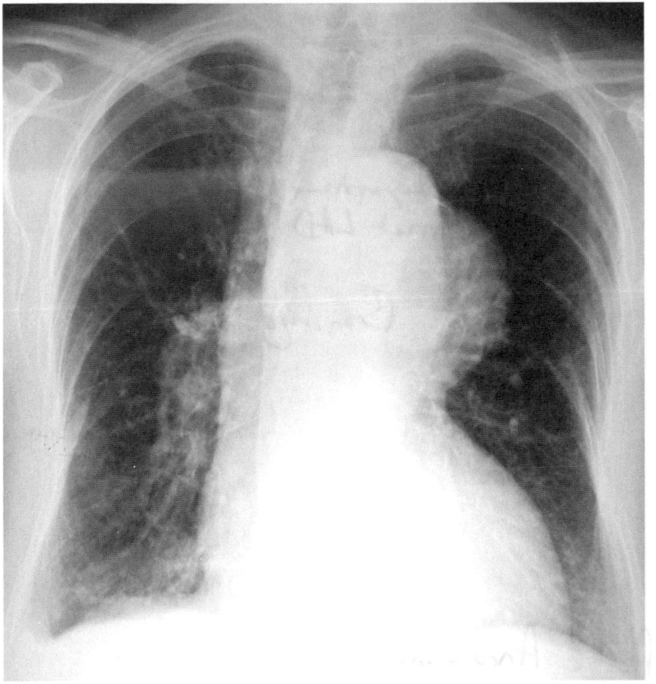

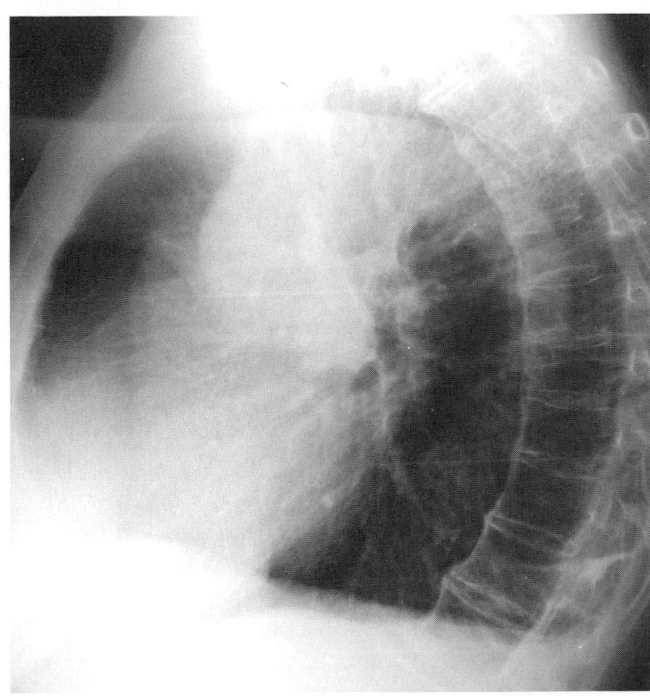

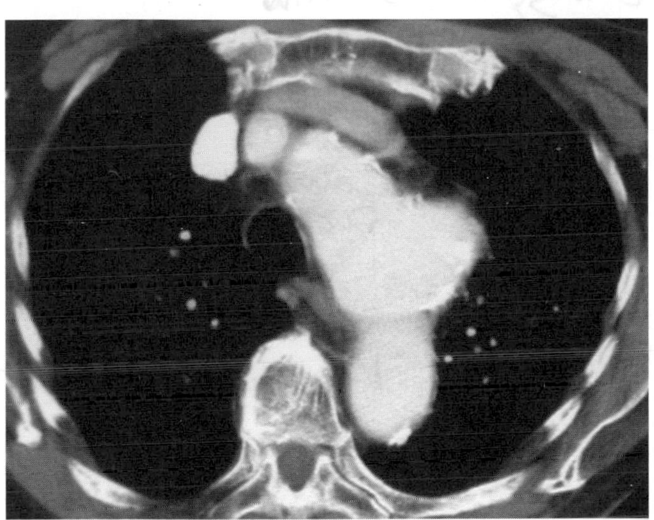

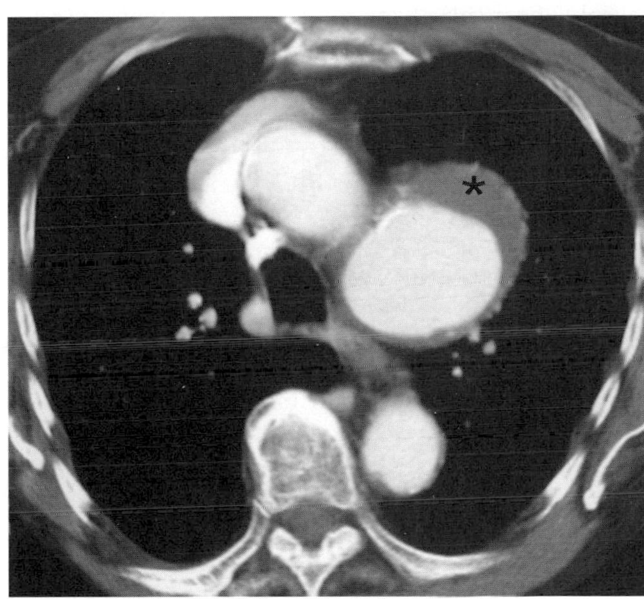

1. What is the differential diagnosis of the mass on the chest radiographs?
2. What is the diagnosis?
3. What is the nonenhancing area (*)?
4. What is the most likely cause of the lesion?

CASE 42

Aortic Arch Aneurysm

1. Bronchogenic cyst, lymphadenopathy, aneurysm of the aortic arch, and pulmonary artery aneurysm are some of the differential considerations.
2. Aneurysm of the aortic arch.
3. Mural thrombus/atherosclerotic plaque.
4. Atherosclerosis.

Reference

Gotway MB, Dawn SK. Thoracic aorta imaging with multislice CT. *Radiol Clin North Am* 41:521–543, 2003.

Cross-Reference

Cardiac Imaging: THE REQUISITES, 2nd edition, pp 368–369, 398–400.

Comment

The chest radiographs demonstrate a well-circumscribed mass that is distinct from the ascending aorta and descending aorta. The CT scan shows a large saccular aneurysm arising from the aortic arch. There is a large amount of organized "mural thrombus" (atherosclerotic plaque) within the aneurysm.

Aortic enlargement is termed an aneurysm when the diameter is more than 5 cm. The maximum diameter of the aorta is an important determinant of the risk of rupture. If the diameter is 6 cm or greater, the risk of rupture in the short term is greater than 30%.

In a true aneurysm of the aorta, all three layers of the aortic wall are intact. In contrast, a false aneurysm results from a focal disruption of one or more layers of the aortic wall and may be contained by the adventitia and surrounding fibrous tissue. On CT and MRI, true aneurysms have wide necks (as in this patient) and false aneurysms have narrow necks. True aneurysms most commonly are secondary to atherosclerosis. Other etiologies include infection, connective tissue disorders such as Marfan syndrome, aortitis, idiopathic cystic medial necrosis, complications of aortic valve disease, and aneurysm of the ductal remnant.

In the imaging assessment of a thoracic aortic aneurysm, the demonstration of mural thrombus is important in patients with peripheral embolization.

Notes

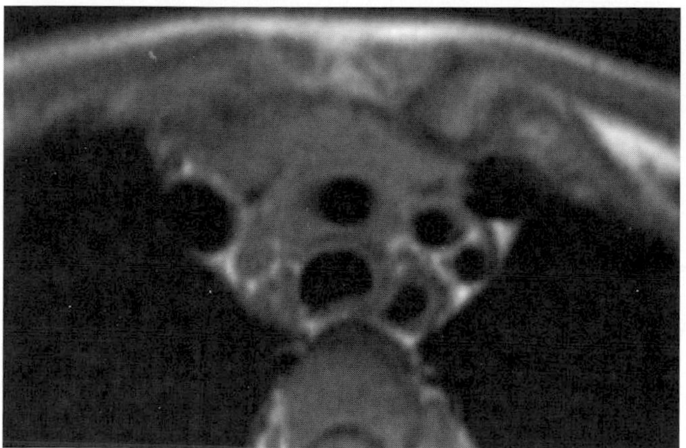

Axial spin-echo MR image.

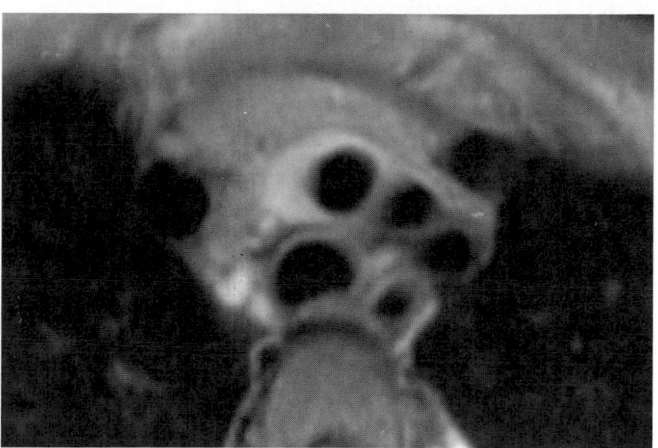

Axial spin-echo postgadolinium MR image with fat saturation.

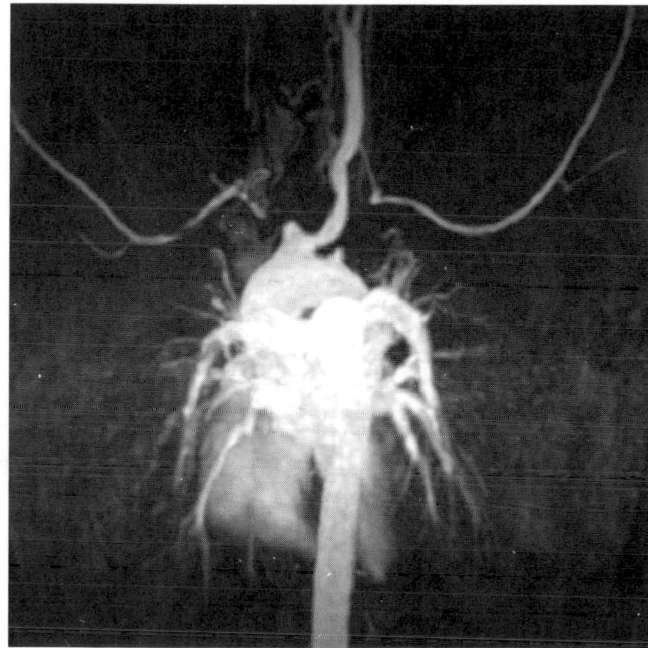

Maximum-intensity projection of gadolinium-enhanced MR angiogram.

1. Which vessels are narrowed?
2. What is the most likely diagnosis in a young woman?
3. Is this disease in the active (inflammatory) phase?
4. What are some of the other thoracic vessels that are commonly involved in this disease?

ANSWERS

CASE 43

Takayasu Arteritis

1. Brachiocephalic, left common carotid, and left subclavian arteries.
2. Takayasu arteritis.
3. Yes.
4. Aorta, right common carotid, subclavian, and pulmonary arteries.

Reference

Gotway MB, Araoz PA, Macedo TA, et al. Imaging findings in Takayasu's arteritis. *AJR Am J Roentgenol* 184:1945–1950, 2005.

Cross-Reference

Cardiac Imaging: THE REQUISITES, 2nd edition, pp 384–387.

Comment

The MRI demonstrates narrowing of the proximal arch vessels. The vessel walls are thickened, and they enhance, indicating the active (inflammatory) phase of arteritis. In a young woman, the most likely diagnosis is Takayasu arteritis.

In Takayasu arteritis, MRI and CT can show stenosis, occlusion, or dilatation of the aorta and its branches, or a combination of all three. Takayasu arteritis is characterized by wall thickening of the aorta and/or arch vessels along with stenosis of the aorta and its branches. Other arteries, such as the pulmonary arteries, can be involved. In patients in the active phase of arteritis, gadolinium-enhanced spin-echo MRI demonstrates wall thickening and enhancement of the involved vessels. Noninvasive imaging with MRI or CT may be particularly valuable in patients with severe stenosis or occlusion of the arch vessels or of the abdominal aorta, because it may be especially difficult to pass an angiography catheter into the thoracic aorta.

Notes

CASE 44

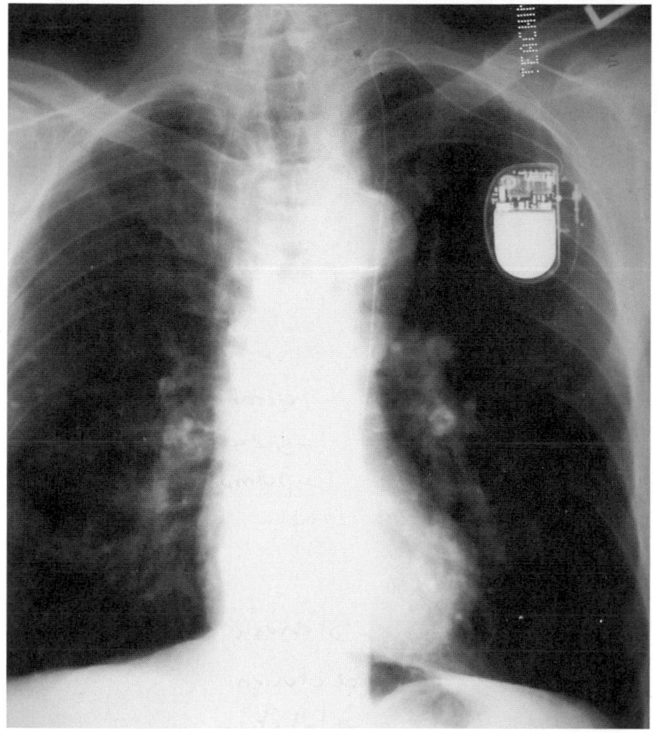

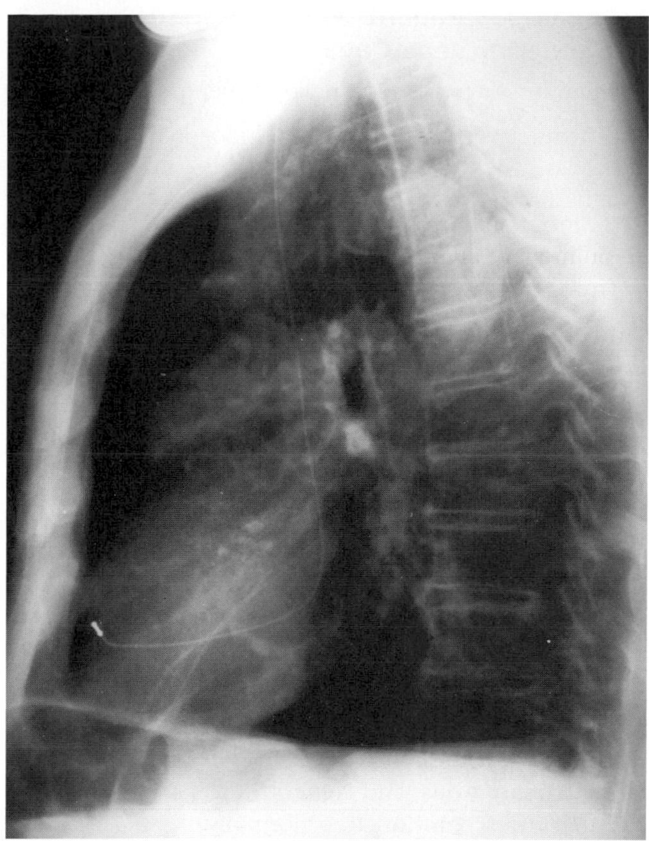

1. Where are the pacemaker lead tips?
2. What is the course of the pacemaker?
3. Can the pacemaker function properly with this course?
4. What arterial system does the coronary sinus drain?

CASE 44

Pacemaker in Patient with Persistent Left Superior Vena Cava

1. Right atrial appendage and right ventricle.
2. Left subclavian artery, left brachiocephalic artery, persistent left superior vena cava, coronary sinus, right atrium, right ventricle.
3. Yes.
4. The coronary arterial system.

Reference

Minniti S, Visentini S, Procacci C. Congenital anomalies of the venae cavae: embryological origin, imaging features and report of three new variants. *Eur Radiol* 12:2040–2055, 2002.

Cross-Reference

Cardiac Imaging: THE REQUISITES, 2nd edition, pp 40–41.

Comment

The chest radiographs demonstrate pacemaker leads traversing the left subclavian vein, left brachiocephalic vein, coronary sinus, and right atrium. Pacemakers that take this course can function normally.

Persistent left superior vena cava results when the left anterior cardinal vein persists after birth. The left brachiocephalic vein drains into the left superior vena cava, which usually connects to the coronary sinus. The coronary sinus may be dilated from the increase in flow, especially if there is no right superior vena cava. Most individuals with a persistent left superior vena cava have a right superior vena cava as well, and their anatomy is otherwise normal. The anomaly may be seen incidentally on a CT scan, or it may come to light after placement of a central venous catheter, pulmonary artery catheter, or a pacemaker.

Notes

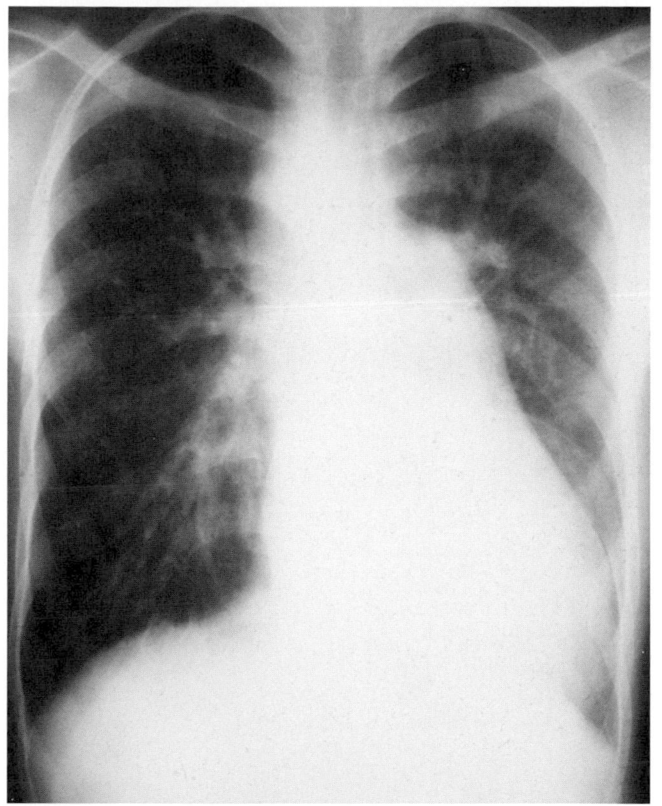

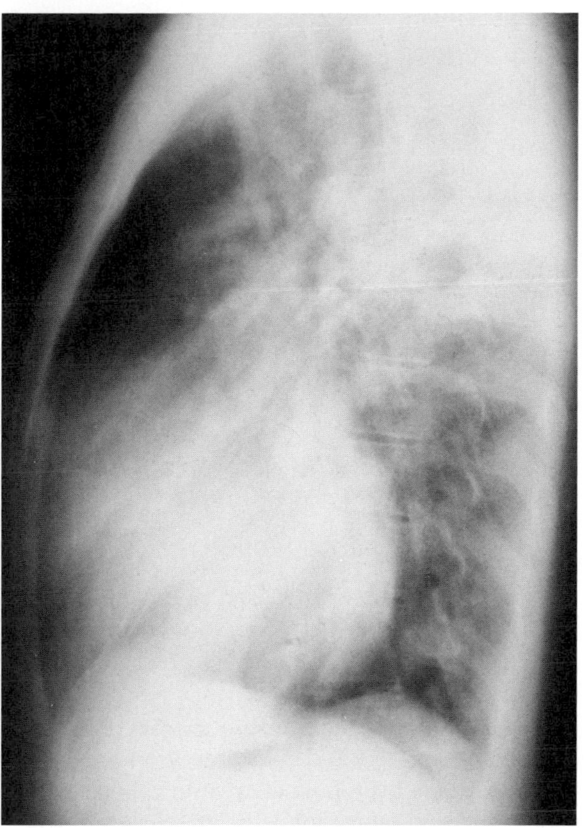

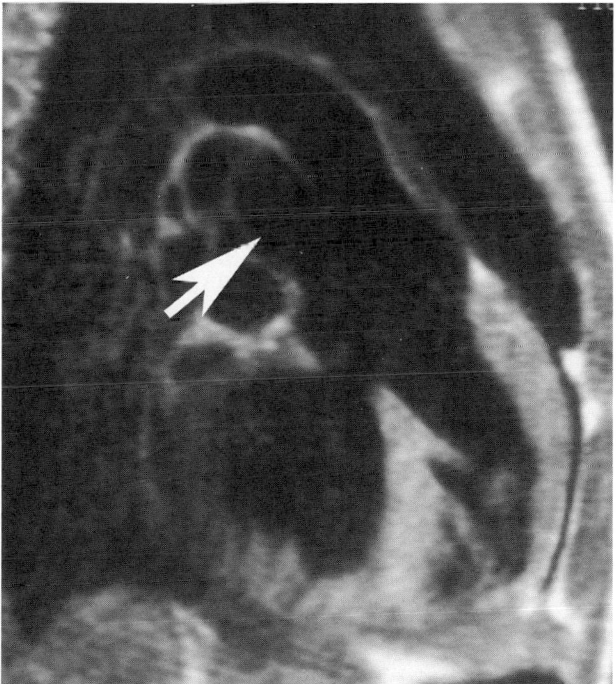

Sagittal spin-echo MR image.

1. Is pulmonary vascularity increased?
2. On which side is the aortic arch located?
3. What structure is indicated by the arrow?
4. In a cyanotic patient, what is the most likely diagnosis?

ANSWERS

CASE 45

Truncus Arteriosus

1. Yes.
2. Right side.
3. Pulmonary artery.
4. Truncus arteriosus.

Reference

Reddy GP, Higgins CB. Magnetic resonance imaging of congenital heart disease: evaluation of morphology and function. *Semin Roentgenol* 38:342–351, 2003.

Cross-Reference

Cardiac Imaging: THE REQUISITES, 2nd edition, pp 310–314.

Comment

The chest radiographs show increased pulmonary vascularity, cardiomegaly, and a right-sided aortic arch. The MR image demonstrates that the pulmonary artery and aorta arise from a common trunk.

Truncus arteriosus is a cyanotic admixture lesion in which the pulmonary artery and aorta arise from a common trunk. There may be a main pulmonary artery, but in some patients the right and left pulmonary arteries arise separately from the common trunk. A ventricular septal defect is present. The truncal valve usually is tricuspid but can have four or more leaflets. Approximately 30% to 35% of patients have a mirror-image right aortic arch.

Plain films show shunt vascularity, cardiomegaly, and frequently a right-sided aortic arch.

Notes

Collett Edwards Classification

1 common origin @ aortic root

2 ascending aorta

3 separate orifices from Ascending Aorta

4 separate origins of (R) + (L) PA from descending aorta

CASE 46

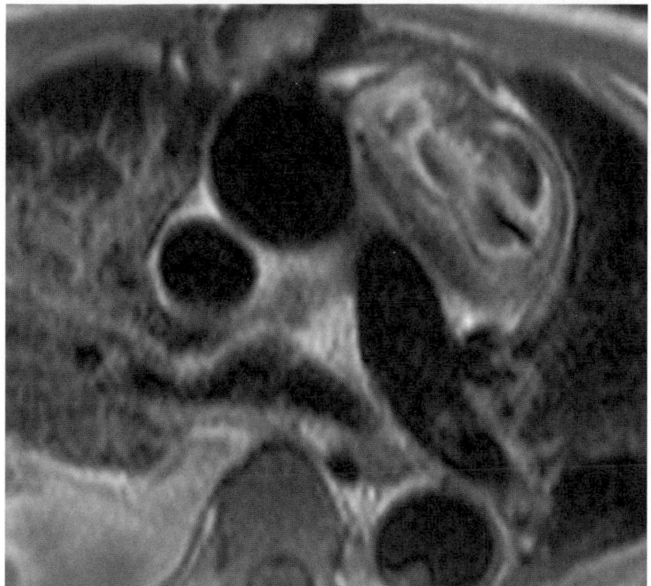
Axial spin-echo MR image.

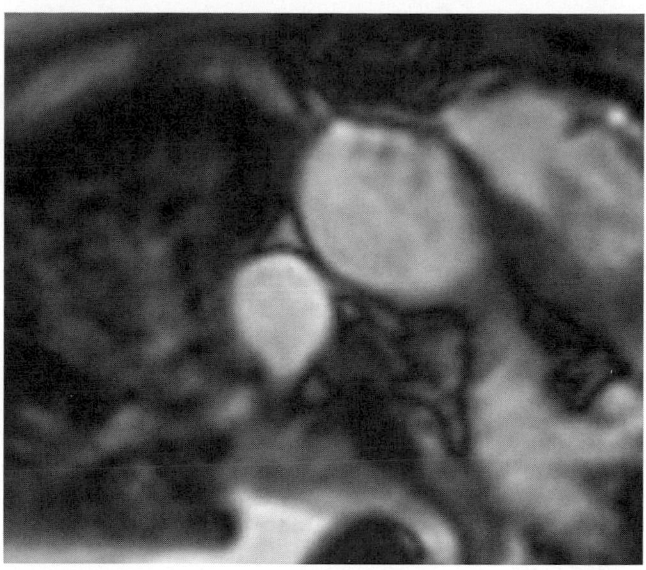
Axial gradient echo cine-MR image.

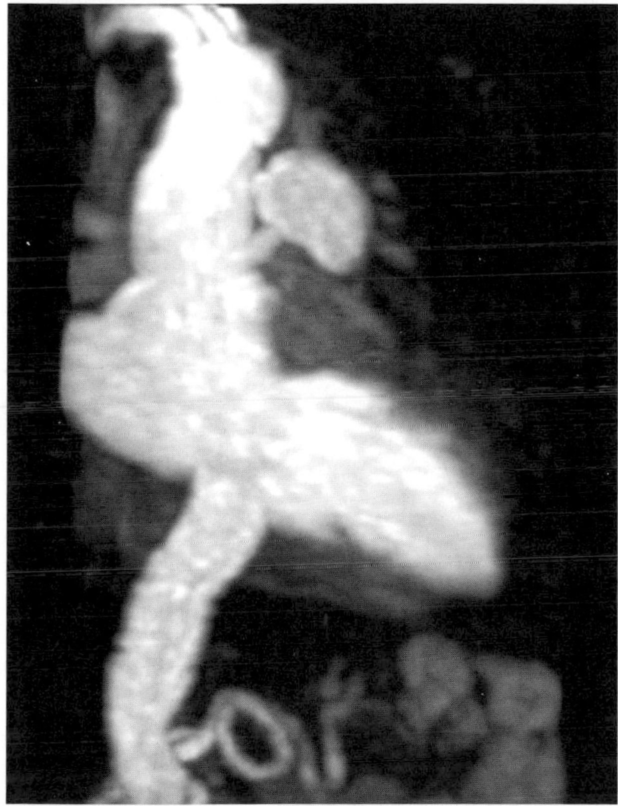
Maximal intensity projection of a gadolinium-enhanced MR angiogram.

1. Where is the mass?
2. Is the mass vascular?
3. This patient has a history of heart surgery. What is the diagnosis?
4. Why is there heterogeneous signal intensity within the mass on the spin-echo (black blood) image?

CASE 46

Aneurysm of Coronary Artery Bypass Graft

1. In the left side of the superior mediastinum.
2. Yes.
3. An aneurysm of a coronary artery bypass graft.
4. There is slow flow within the aneurysm.

Reference

Reddy GP, Steiner RM. Aneurysm of saphenous vein coronary bypass graft: diagnosis by computed tomography. *J Thorac Imaging* 14:147–149, 1999.

Cross-Reference

Cardiac Imaging: THE REQUISITES, 2nd edition, pp 226–227.

Comment

The MR image demonstrates a mass in the superior mediastinum, just to the left of the ascending aorta. The maximum-intensity projection image of the contrast-enhanced MR angiogram during the systemic arterial phase shows that the mass is connected to the aorta and that it is filled with contrast agent. This is an aneurysm of a saphenous vein coronary artery bypass graft.

Aneurysms of coronary artery bypass grafts are rare. They occur more frequently in saphenous vein grafts than in internal mammary artery grafts. A pseudo-aneurysm can occur at the anastomotic site; true aneurysms occur within the graft and are secondary to atherosclerosis. Patients may require reoperation for aneurysm repair.

Plain films can show a round or oval mediastinal mass. Contrast-enhanced CT or MR angiography can establish the diagnosis.

Notes

CASE 47

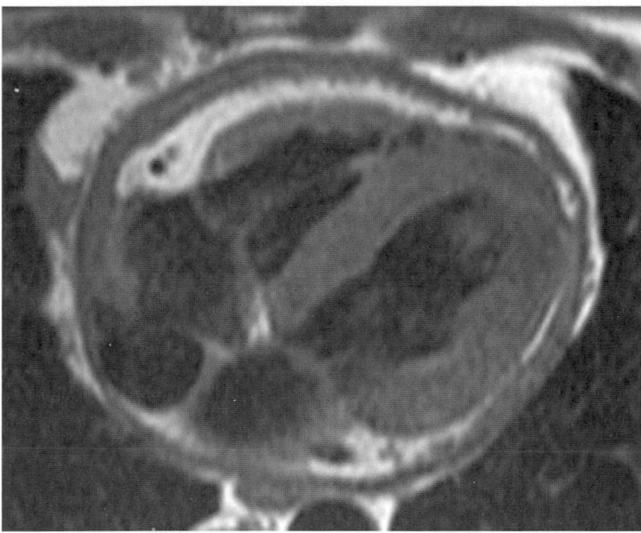

Axial spin-echo MR image.

1. What is the pericardial abnormality?
2. What are the MRI findings of constrictive pericarditis?
3. Does MRI alone establish the diagnosis of constrictive pericarditis?
4. What are the most common causes of constrictive pericarditis in the United States?

CASE 48

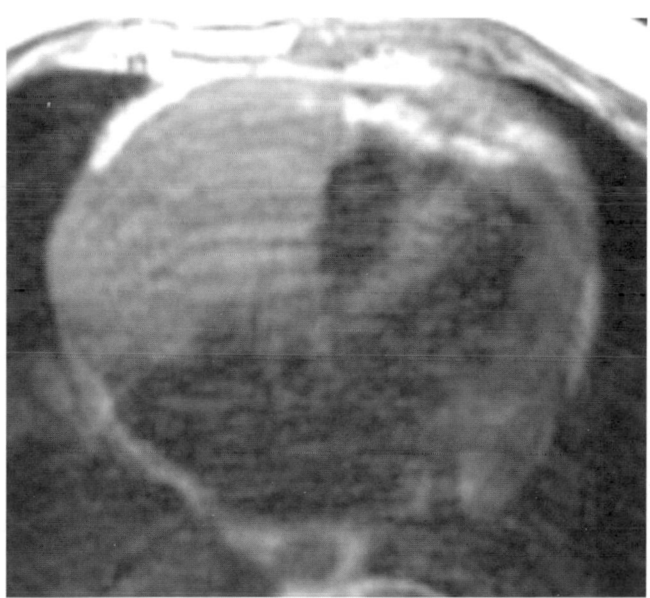

Axial spin-echo MR image.

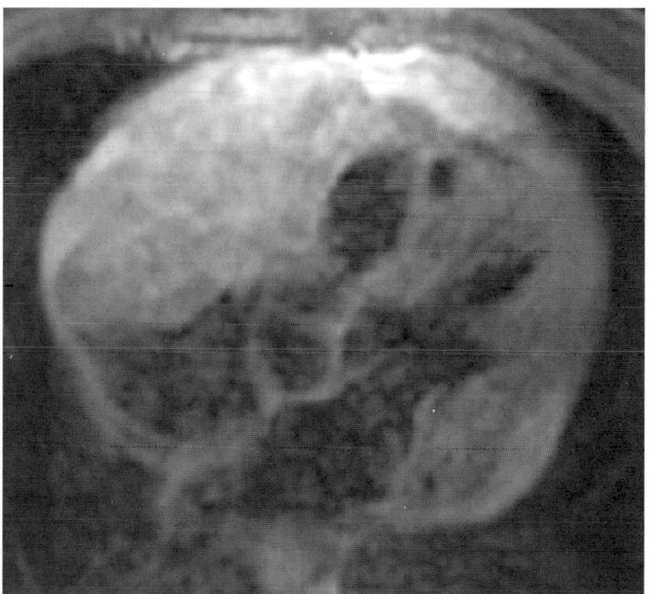

Axial spin-echo postgadolinium MR image with fat saturation.

1. How many chambers are involved?
2. Is the mass infiltrative?
3. Is the mass benign or malignant?
4. What is the most likely diagnosis?

ANSWERS

CASE 47

Constrictive Pericarditis

1. Thickening.
2. Pericardial thickening (≥4 mm) and diastolic dysfunction of the interventricular septum (septal bounce).
3. No. Clinical information is necessary to confirm that the patient has constrictive/restrictive physiology.
4. Cardiac surgery, radiation therapy, uremic pericarditis, viral pericarditis, tuberculous pericarditis.

Reference

Wang ZJ, Reddy GP, Gotway MB, Yeh BM, Hetts SW, Higgins CB. CT and MR imaging of pericardial disease. *Radiographics* 23(Special Issue):S167–S180, 2003.

Cross-Reference

Cardiac Imaging: THE REQUISITES, 2nd edition, pp 253–256.

Comment

Constrictive pericarditis occurs when limitation in diastolic ventricular filling leads to equalization of atrial and ventricular pressure, which is known as constrictive/restrictive physiology. Patients have symptoms similar to those of congestive heart failure. Physical examination may demonstrate the classic Kussmaul sign, which is the paradoxical elevation of jugular venous pressure on inspiration. Causes of constrictive pericarditis include open heart surgery, radiation therapy, uremic pericarditis, viral pericarditis, and (less commonly in industrialized countries) tuberculous pericarditis.

Constrictive pericarditis and restrictive cardiomyopathy have similar clinical presentations and findings on echocardiography and cardiac catheterization. However, it is important to differentiate between these two diseases because patients with constrictive disease usually benefit from pericardiectomy, whereas restrictive cardiomyopathy has a poor prognosis and must be managed medically or with heart transplantation.

In the clinical setting of constrictive/restrictive physiology, pericardial thickening (≥4 mm) as demonstrated on MRI can establish the diagnosis of constrictive pericarditis. Diastolic septal dysfunction (septal bounce) on cine-MRI is another key finding. Ancillary findings may be present, including dilatation of the inferior vena cava, hepatic veins, and right atrium, with a narrow, tubular right ventricle.

It is important to remember that pericardial thickening can occur in the absence of constrictive physiology. Therefore, the diagnosis of constrictive pericarditis can be established only in the appropriate clinical setting of constrictive/restrictive physiology.

Notes

CASE 48

Cardiac Lymphoma

1. Two.
2. Yes.
3. Malignant.
4. Secondary tumor.

Reference

Restrepo CS, Largoza A, Lemos DF, et al. CT and MR imaging findings of malignant cardiac tumors. *Curr Probl Diagn Radiol* 34:1–11, 2005.

Cross-Reference

Cardiac Imaging: THE REQUISITES, 2nd edition, pp 261, 270.

Comment

The MR image depicts a large, infiltrating mass involving the right atrium and right ventricle. These findings indicate a malignant tumor. When the patient has a known malignant neoplasm elsewhere in the body, the most likely diagnosis is secondary tumor involvement of the heart. Definitive diagnosis can be achieved by endomyocardial or open biopsy. This patient had non-Hodgkin lymphoma involving the mediastinum and extending into the heart.

Approximately 98% of cardiac tumors are secondary tumors, most commonly from direct extension (lymphoma or metastatic breast or lung carcinoma) or hematogenous spread (melanoma, lung or breast carcinoma). In patients with renal cell carcinoma, the tumor can enter the right atrium via the inferior vena cava.

MRI can be used to demonstrate tumor size and location as well as cardiac function. Contrast-enhanced sequences can delineate tumor margins and invasion into adjacent structures. It is important to remember that the presence of enhancement does not signify malignancy; benign tumors also enhance.

Notes

CASE 49

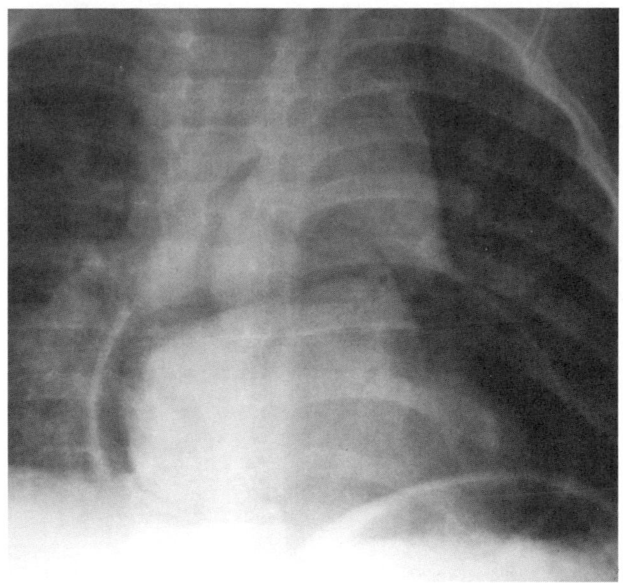

1. What is the finding?
2. What are some etiologies for this finding?
3. How can barotrauma cause this finding?
4. How can a malignant neoplasm cause this finding?

CASE 50

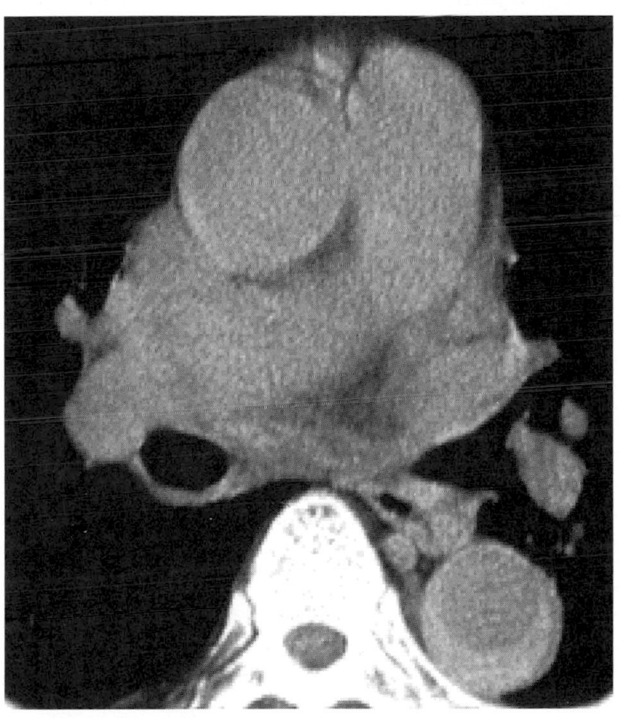

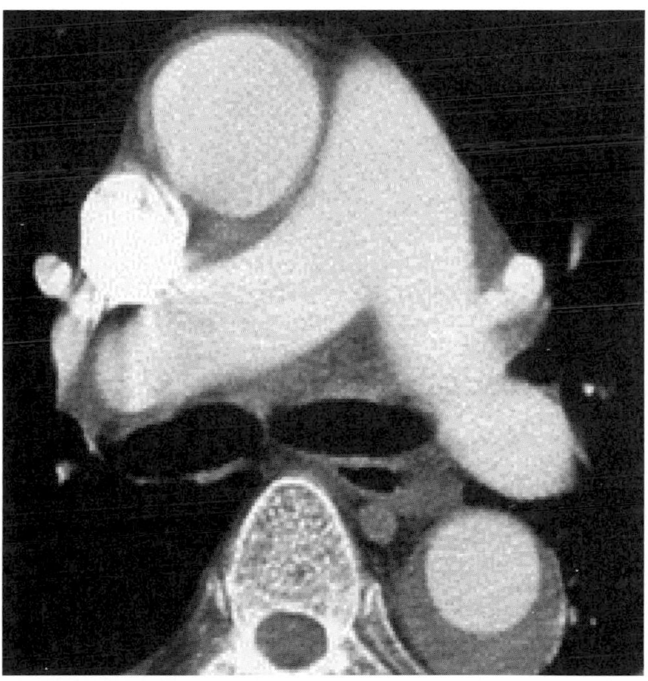

1. What is the high-density material in the aortic wall?
2. What is the diagnosis?
3. Would this be classified as Stanford type A or type B?
4. Does this lesion require surgery?

CASE 49

Pneumopericardium

1. Pneumopericardium; air in the pericardial space.
2. Trauma, iatrogenic cause (pericardiocentesis, surgery, barotrauma), esophageal-pericardial fistula, malignancy.
3. Interstitial air dissects along the pulmonary vessels. This occurs relatively commonly in children but is rare in adults except after cardiac surgery or pericardial instrumentation.
4. Usually secondary to a fistula such as an esophageal-pericardial fistula.

References

Trotman-Dickenson B. Radiology in the intensive care unit (part 2). *J Intensive Care Med* 18:239–252, 2003.

Song H, Choi YW, Jang IS, Jeon SC, et al. Pericardium: anatomy and spectrum of disease on computed tomography. *Curr Probl Diagn Radiol* 31:198–209, 2002.

Comment

This infant has a large air collection in the pericardial space. Air is also noted outlining the pericardial recesses.

Pneumopericardium is most commonly posttraumatic or iatrogenic. After pericardiocentesis, a small amount of air is frequently seen in the pericardium, but a large pneumopericardium is unusual. In infants, barotrauma can result in a large pneumopericardium. In this setting, the pneumopericardium is usually self-limiting and resolves spontaneously.

In rare instances, an esophageal-pericardial fistula can develop, sometimes secondary to a malignant tumor. In this setting, patients may have a hydropneumopericardium.

Notes

Pneumopericardium
DDx: - Trauma
- Iatrogenic - Pericardiocentesis
- Surgery
- Esophageal Pericardial Fistula

c Peds: Barotrauma c air dissecting along the pulmonary vessels

c Malignancy ⇒ 2° Fistula - esophageal-pericardial
- bronchial pericardial

CASE 50

Intramural Hematoma—Stanford Type B

1. Blood (hematoma).
2. Intramural hematoma.
3. Stanford type B. The hematoma involves the descending aorta only.
4. No; type B intramural hematomas can be managed medically.

Reference

Gotway MB, Dawn SK. Thoracic aorta imaging with multislice CT. *Radiol Clin North Am* 41:521–543, 2003.

Cross-Reference

Cardiac Imaging: THE REQUISITES, 2nd edition, pp 402–406.

Comment

The CT scan demonstrates blood in the aortic wall, manifested by wall thickening and high density of the wall.

An intramural hematoma is most commonly caused by rupture of the vasa vasorum, the arteries that supply the aortic wall. The ruptured vessels bleed into the aortic wall, which can result in an intimal tear and separation of the wall—a frank dissection. If the intima does not separate, then an intramural hematoma remains. The intramural hematoma may remain localized, or it can extend along the wall in an antegrade or a retrograde direction or rarely rupture through the adventitia. Intramural hematoma can be considered to be a type of dissection, and treatment is similar to that of a frank dissection. Stanford type B intramural hematomas are usually managed medically, and type A hematomas may need to be treated surgically.

CT shows characteristic high-density thickening of the aortic wall. On MRI, the signal intensity is intermediate to high on spin-echo sequences. Relying solely on gadolinium-enhanced MRA can be risky in the setting of dissection because an intramural hematoma can be overlooked on this sequence.

Notes

CASE 51

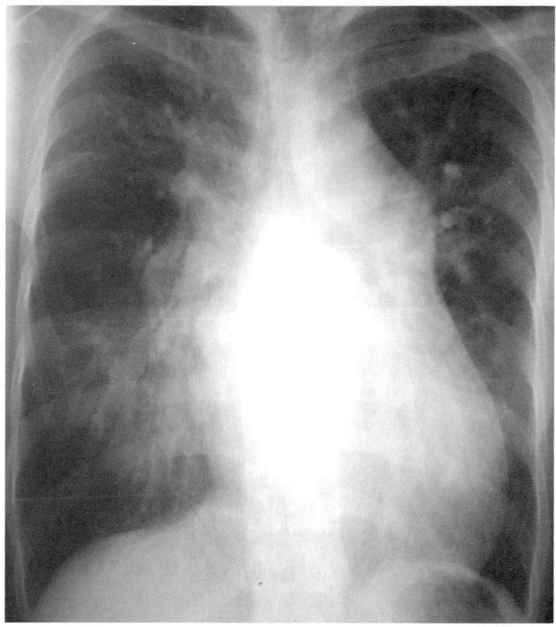

1. Is pulmonary vascularity increased or decreased?
2. Is the left atrium enlarged?
3. Is the aortic arch normal?
4. In an acyanotic patient, what is the most likely diagnosis?

CASE 52

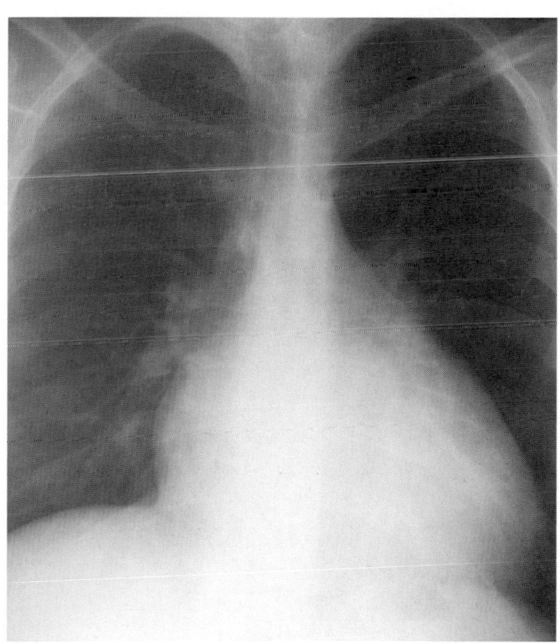

1. What is the most common cause of dilated cardiomyopathy?
2. In a young adult, what are some causes of dilated cardiomyopathy?
3. What is the clinical hallmark of dilated cardiomyopathy?
4. How is dilated cardiomyopathy managed?

ANSWERS

CASE 51

Patent Ductus Arteriosus

1. Increased.
2. Yes.
3. No; it is enlarged.
4. Patent ductus arteriosus.

Reference

Steiner RM, Reddy GP, Flicker S. Congenital cardiovascular disease in the adult patient: imaging update. *J Thorac Imaging* 17:1–17, 2002.

Cross-Reference

Cardiac Imaging: THE REQUISITES, 2nd edition, pp 334–337.

Comment

The chest radiograph shows enlargement of the left atrium and aortic arch. Pulmonary vascularity is increased. In an acyanotic patient, the most likely diagnosis is patent ductus arteriosus.

In the fetus, the ductus arteriosus is a widely patent vessel that connects the proximal descending aorta to the main or left pulmonary artery, allowing the output of the right ventricle to bypass the lungs. The ductus usually closes shortly after birth as a result of the rise in the partial pressure of oxygen in the circulation. If the ductus does not close, indomethacin can be administered in the first week of life, especially in premature infants. If the ductus remains patent, pulmonary hypertension can develop. In the absence of a coexisting anomaly, the ductus should be closed by surgical ligation or by transcatheter coil embolization.

Notes

CXR: - enlarged (L) Atrium
- enlarged Aortic Knob
- ↑ Vascularity

Acyanotic Pt ⇒ PDA

- To close PDA in 1st week of life ⇒ Indomethacin

CASE 52

Dilated Cardiomyopathy

1. Ischemic heart disease.
2. It can be idiopathic or secondary to alcoholism, hypertension, viral diseases, diabetes, or toxins.
3. Left ventricular failure.
4. By management of ventricular failure. Heart transplantation is the definitive treatment.

Reference

Mistry DJ, Kramer CM. Imaging of cardiopulmonary diseases. *Clin Sports Med* 22:197–212, 2003.

Cross-Reference

Cardiac Imaging: THE REQUISITES, 2nd edition, pp 271–272.

Comment

The chest radiograph demonstrates generalized enlargement of the cardiac silhouette. In a young adult, dilated cardiomyopathy should be considered. The differential diagnosis would include pericardial effusion.

Dilated cardiomyopathy is characterized by failure and enlargement of the left ventricle or both ventricles. The ventricular contractile function is diminished. Treatment involves management of cardiac failure. Patients may be eligible for heart transplantation, which is the definitive treatment.

Notes

CASE 53

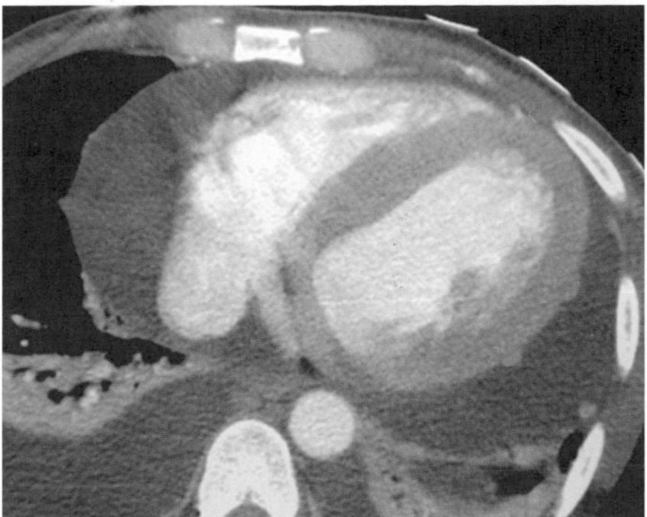

Axial spin-echo MR image.

1. Is there a pericardial effusion?
2. Does the pericardium enhance?
3. Are there pericardial nodules?
4. The patient has a history of breast carcinoma. What is the most likely diagnosis?

CASE 54

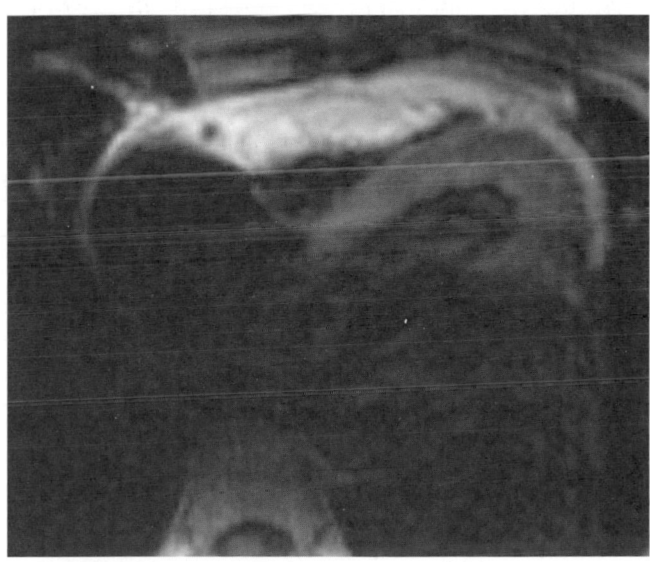

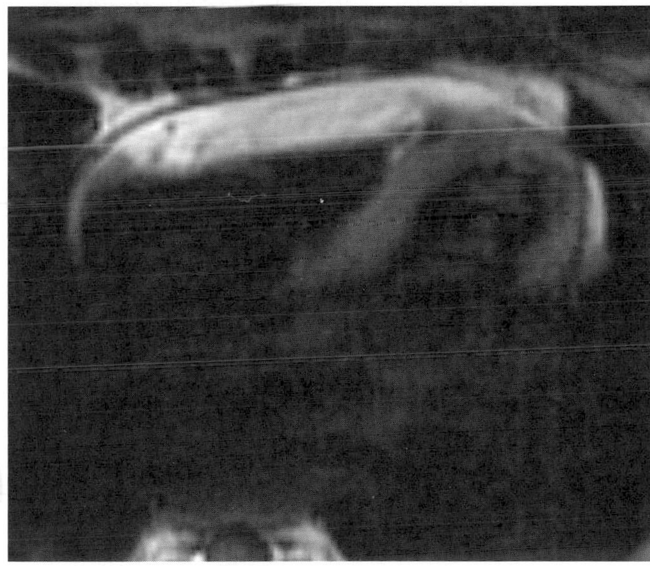

Axial spin-echo MR images.

1. What is the abnormality of the right ventricle?
2. The patient's brother died suddenly during exercise. Autopsy demonstrated gross fat in the right ventricular myocardium. What is the most likely diagnosis?
3. What are some common presenting signs of this disease?
4. Why does endomyocardial biopsy have low sensitivity for this disease?

ANSWERS

CASE 53

Pericardial Metastasis

1. Yes.
2. Yes.
3. Yes.
4. Metastasis.

Reference

Wang ZJ, Reddy GP, Gotway MB, Yeh BM, Hetts SW, Higgins CB. CT and MR imaging of pericardial disease. *Radiographics* 23(Special Issue):S167–S180, 2003.

Cross-Reference

Cardiac Imaging: THE REQUISITES, 2nd edition, p 261.

Comment

This patient with a history of breast carcinoma has a pericardial effusion as well as enhancement and nodular thickening of the pericardium, consistent with metastasis.

Pericardial metastases are much more common than primary neoplasms of the pericardium. Tumor can seed the pericardium via lymphatic or hematogenous dissemination or invade the pericardium directly from the lung or mediastinum. Carcinomas of the breast and lung are the most common neoplasms to involve the pericardium, followed by lymphomas and melanomas. Pericardial metastasis is suggested on CT or MRI by the presence of effusion with an irregularly thickened, nodular pericardium or the actual demonstration of a pericardial mass. The pericardial effusion may be hemorrhagic, which produces high signal intensity on spin-echo MRI. Malignant disease usually enhances following the administration of contrast agent.

Notes

CASE 54

Arrhythmogenic Right Ventricular Dysplasia

1. Fatty infiltration of the myocardium.
2. Arrhythmogenic right ventricular dysplasia.
3. Right ventricular tachyarrhythmia, syncope, sudden death (cardiac arrest).
4. Because the right ventricle might not be uniformly affected, endomyocardial biopsy might not sample the affected areas.

Reference

Bremerich J, Pater S, Buser PT. Magnetic resonance imaging of acquired heart disease: evaluation of structure. *Semin Roentgenol* 38:314–319, 2003.

Cross-Reference

Cardiac Imaging: THE REQUISITES, 2nd edition, pp 277–280.

Comment

Arrhythmogenic right ventricular dysplasia usually presents as recurrent ventricular tachycardia originating from a site in the right ventricle. The pathologic process is replacement of the right ventricular myocardium by fat or fibrous tissue.

MRI by itself cannot establish the diagnosis. The diagnosis of right ventricular dysplasia is made by clinical, electrophysiologic, echocardiographic, and MRI findings. Patients may have a family history of right ventricular dysplasia or of sudden death. They usually demonstrate right ventricular tachyarrhythmia, syncope, or cardiac arrest.

Spin-echo MR images can display transmural fat or islands of fat in the right ventricular myocardium. Other supportive features are focal or generalized wall thinning of the right ventricular free wall, often with a focal aneurysm of the free wall. On cine-MRI, there should be dyskinesis of the abnormal segment of the right ventricle.

Notes

ARVD signs/Sx: (R) Vent Tachyarrhythmia
Syncope
Cardiac arrest
↳ Problem: pathologically > Fatty infiltration of the myocardium
- Dx > Clinical
Imaging - suggestive

CASE 55

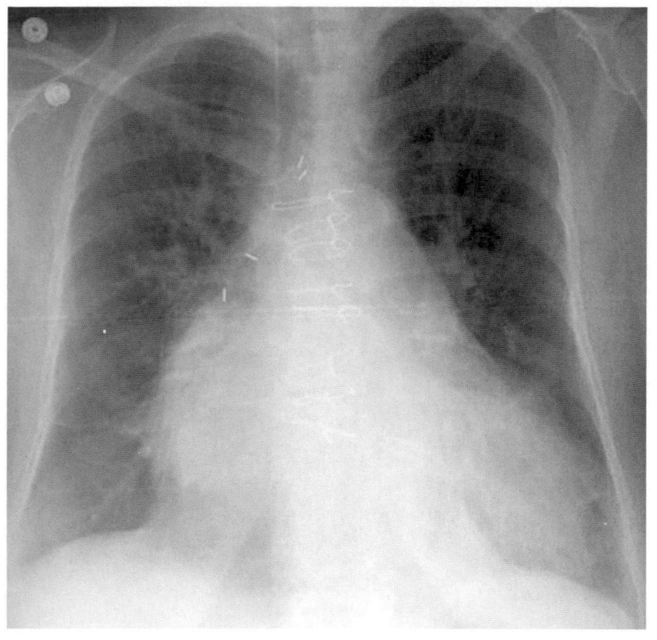

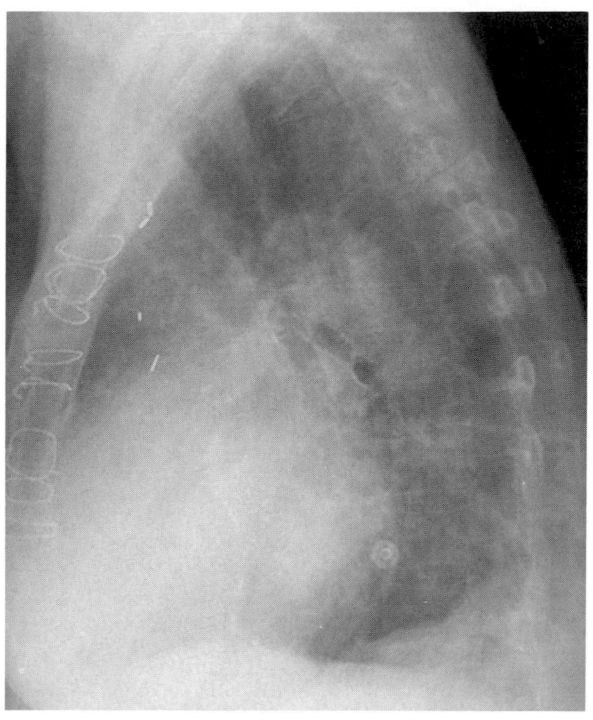

1. Which valvular dysfunction is caused by mitral valve prolapse?
2. Which components of the mitral apparatus are involved in valve prolapse?
3. Which connective tissue disorder is associated with mitral valve prolapse?
4. What is the angiographic hallmark of mitral valve prolapse?

CASE 56

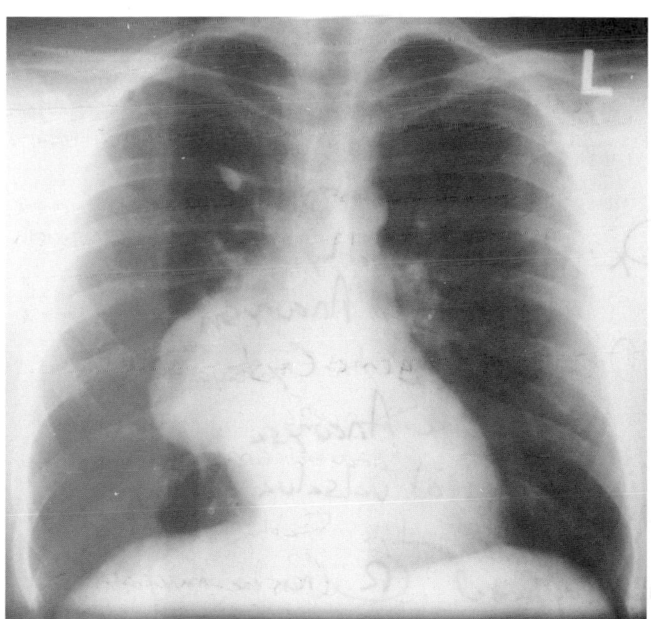

1. What is the differential diagnosis?
2. What is the cause of a sinus of Valsalva aneurysm?
3. What valvular lesion is associated with this lesion?
4. What type of septal defect is associated with this abnormality?

CASE 55

Mitral Valve Prolapse

1. Mitral regurgitation.
2. All components can be involved.
3. Marfan syndrome.
4. The valve leaflets pass behind the plane of the annulus into the left atrium.

Reference

Bonow RO, Cheitlin MD, Crawford MH, Douglas PS. Task Force 3: valvular heart disease. *J Am Coll Cardiol* 45:1334–1340, 2005.

Cross-Reference

Cardiac Imaging: THE REQUISITES, 2nd edition, pp 56–57.

Comment

Mitral valve prolapse can involve all components of the mitral apparatus. Mitral prolapse has a 5% incidence in the general population. In Marfan syndrome, congenital prolapse occurs in the mitral and tricuspid valves because the valve leaflets are redundant. If prolapse is mild, the heart may be normal. More severe prolapse may result in severe regurgitation, subacute bacterial endocarditis, chest pain, or rarely death. Geometric distortion of the left ventricle can cause moderate mitral prolapse.

Mitral prolapse can be identified on echocardiography. Echocardiography can be used to grade the severity of prolapse and the presence and degree of regurgitation. The angiographic hallmark of mitral prolapse is the passage of the leaflets behind the plane of the annulus into the left atrium.

Notes

CASE 56

Sinus of Valsalva Aneurysm

1. Lymphadenopathy, pulmonary artery aneurysm, bronchogenic cyst, aortic aneurysm, sinus of Valsalva aneurysm.
2. It usually results from congenital weakness at the junction of the aorta and the valve.
3. Aortic regurgitation.
4. Supracristal ventricular septal defect.

Reference

Goldberg N, Krasnow N. Sinus of Valsalva aneurysms. *Clin Cardiol* 13:831–836, 1990.

Cross-Reference

Cardiac Imaging: THE REQUISITES, 2nd edition, pp 382–383.

Comment

The chest radiograph shows a mass arising from the right side of the mediastinum.

Sinus of Valsalva aneurysms usually result from congenital weakness at the junction of the aortic media and the annulus fibrosis of the valve. They most frequently arise from the right or noncoronary sinuses. Aneurysms of the right coronary sinus rupture into the right atrium or ventricle, and aneurysms of the noncoronary sinus rupture into the right atrium. Sinus of Valsalva aneurysms are associated with aortic regurgitation. They can occur in patients who have a supracristal ventricular septal defect.

On imaging examinations, a sinus of Valsalva aneurysm presents as a focal dilation of one sinus of Valsalva, in contrast to the generalized aortic root dilation seen in annuloaortic ectasia.

Notes

CASE 57

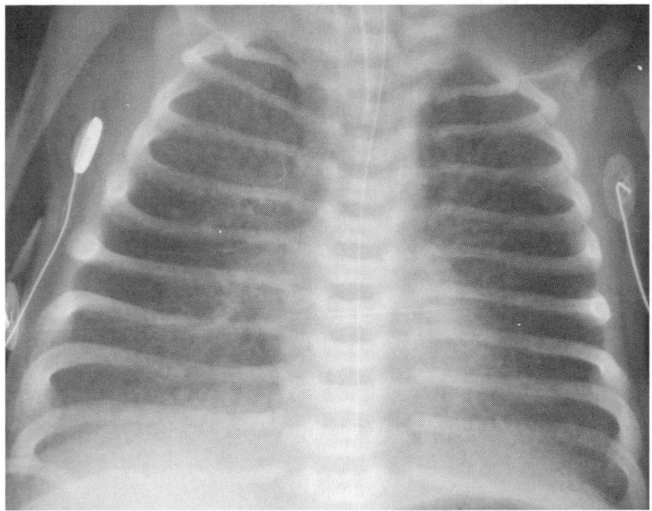

1. Does this patient have pulmonary edema?
2. Is the heart enlarged?
3. The infant was one day old. What is the most likely diagnosis?
4. Would you expect this baby to be cyanotic?

CASE 58

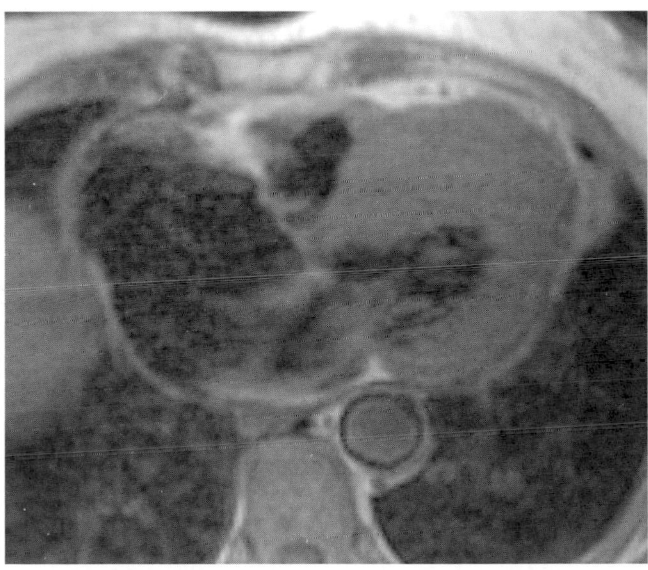

Axial spin-echo MR image.

1. Which part of the left ventricle is abnormal?
2. How is this condition differentiated from a tumor?
3. What is the most likely diagnosis?
4. What is the most common distribution of myocardial thickening in this disease?

CASE 57

Total Anomalous Pulmonary Venous Connection—Type III (Connection below Diaphragm)

1. Yes.
2. No.
3. Total anomalous pulmonary venous connection: type III (connection below diaphragm).
4. Yes.

Reference

Higgins CB. Radiography of congenital heart disease. In Webb WR, Higgins CB, editors: *Thoracic imaging: pulmonary and cardiovascular radiology*. Philadelphia, 2005, Lippincott Williams & Wilkins, pp 679–706.

Cross-Reference

Cardiac Imaging: THE REQUISITES, 2nd edition, pp 316–319.

Comment

The chest radiograph demonstrates pulmonary edema. The heart size is normal. In a one-day-old infant, the most likely diagnosis is total anomalous pulmonary venous connection-type III (connection below diaphragm).

In this anomaly, all the pulmonary veins drain into the systemic veins or directly into the right atrium. In the supracardiac type (I), the enlarged mediastinal veins cause the "snowman heart" appearance. In the cardiac type (II), the pulmonary veins drain into the coronary sinus or right atrium. In the infracardiac type (III), the veins connect to the portal vein, hepatic vein, or ductus venosus. Venous flow is obstructed by the passage of the pulmonary veins across the esophageal hiatus, leading to pulmonary congestion and edema without cardiac enlargement.

Notes

CASE 58

Hypertrophic Cardiomyopathy

1. Septum.
2. The contrast-enhanced image would show marked enhancement if there was a tumor in the septum.
3. Hypertrophic cardiomyopathy.
4. Asymmetric septal hypertrophy.

Reference

Soler R, Rodriguez E, Remuinan C, Bello MJ, Diaz A. Magnetic resonance imaging of primary cardiomyopathies. *J Comput Assist Tomogr* 27:724–734, 2003.

Cross-Reference

Cardiac Imaging: THE REQUISITES, 2nd edition, pp 272–275.

Comment

Hypertrophic cardiomyopathy (HCM) is inherited as an autosomal dominant trait with variable penetrance. Patients have a variable clinical presentation: they may be asymptomatic or they may have atrial fibrillation, heart failure, syncope, or even sudden cardiac death, which is the leading cause of mortality in these patients. Asymmetric hypertrophy of the ventricular septum accounts for 90% of cases of HCM. Other patterns exhibit right ventricular, left ventricular, septal, apical, mid-ventricular, or concentric distribution. Patients with heart failure secondary to significant septal hypertrophy and left ventricular outflow obstruction can be treated with septal myectomy or percutaneous transluminal septal myocardial ablation with ethanol.

MRI can provide anatomic and functional information in HCM and can be most useful when the diagnosis is in question, when invasive therapy is being considered, or when clinical concern requires more thorough assessment than that provided by echocardiography. MRI can be used to identify the distribution of thickened myocardium and to calculate left ventricular mass. To differentiate HCM from a septal neoplasm, gadolinium-chelate contrast agent is administered intravenously. A neoplasm will enhance markedly, whereas septal hypertrophic myocardium enhances only slightly. MRI also can be used for functional evaluation of left ventricular outflow tract obstruction and myocardial perfusion and viability.

Notes

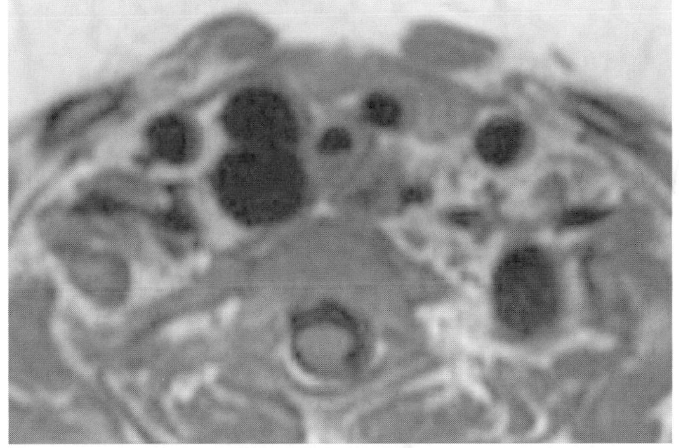

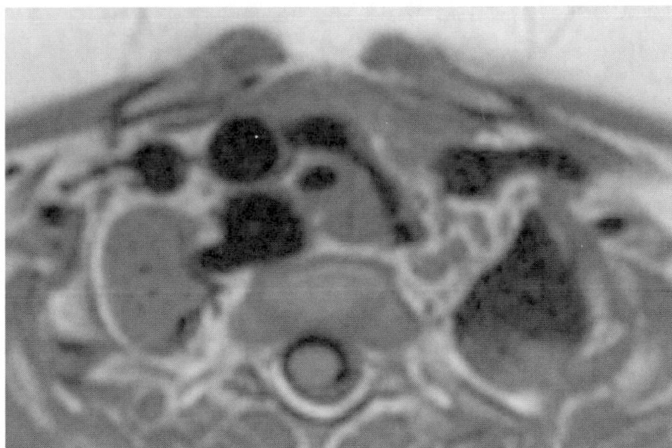

Axial spin-echo MR images.

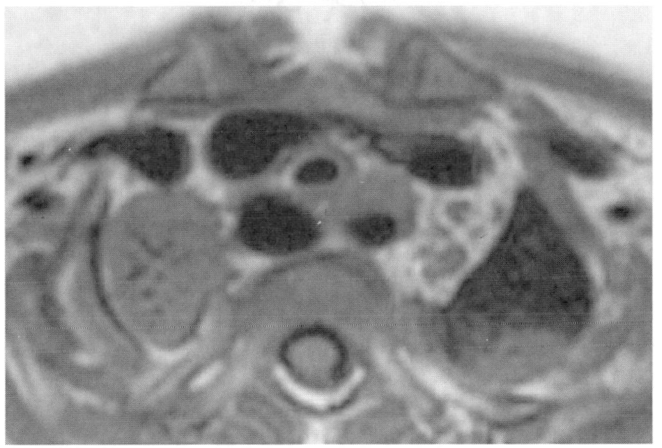

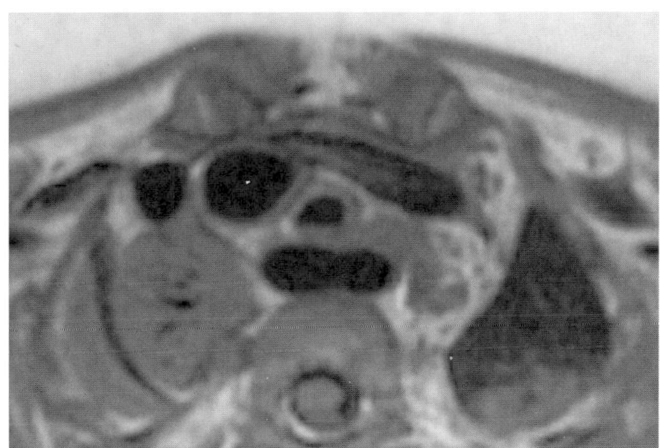

1. What is the anomaly?
2. Does this anomaly represent a vascular ring?
3. What are some common symptoms of this lesion?
4. Where does the anomalous vessel pass with respect to the esophagus?

CASE 59

Double Aortic Arch

1. Double aortic arch.
2. Yes.
3. Wheezing, dyspnea, dysphagia.
4. Posterior to the esophagus.

Reference

Reddy GP, Higgins CB. Magnetic resonance imaging of congenital heart disease: evaluation of morphology and function. *Semin Roentgenol* 38:342–351, 2003.

Cross-Reference

Cardiac Imaging: THE REQUISITES, 2nd edition, pp 407–408.

Comment

The MRI demonstrates a double aortic arch. The right arch is larger and higher than the left arch. Note the compression of the trachea.

A double aortic arch is the most common type of vascular ring. It occurs when both fourth fetal arches persist. If there is partial involution of one of the arches, then the double arch will be incomplete. The right arch is usually higher and larger than the left. The aorta usually descends on the left.

The vascular ring compresses the trachea and esophagus to a variable extent. The most common symptoms are wheezing, dyspnea, and dysphagia, and patients often have these symptoms during early childhood.

MRI and CT can depict the vascular anatomy and the compression of the trachea and esophagus. Cine-MRI has the added advantage of demonstrating dynamic compression of the trachea during pulsation of the aorta and arch vessels. MRI or CT can be used for preoperative evaluation of the sizes of the two arches. Typically the smaller arch is surgically ligated.

Notes

CASE 60

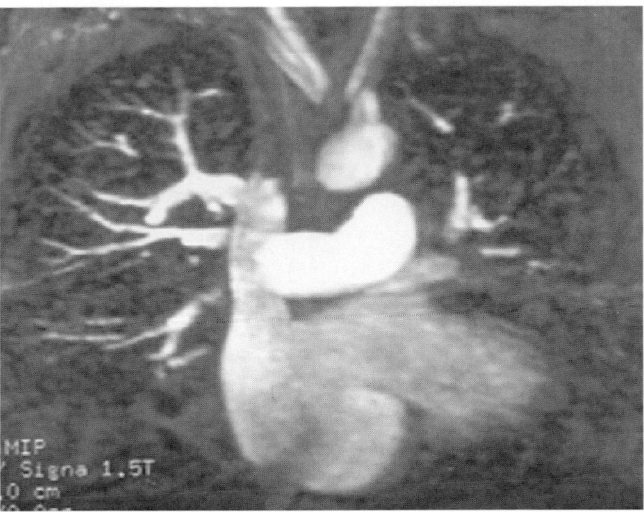

Gadolinium-enhanced MR angiogram.

1. What is the anomaly?
2. Does this anomaly represent a left-to-right shunt or a right-to-left shunt?
3. Is the shunt at the atrial level or postatrial level?
4. What type of atrial septal defect is most commonly associated with the anomaly?

CASE 61

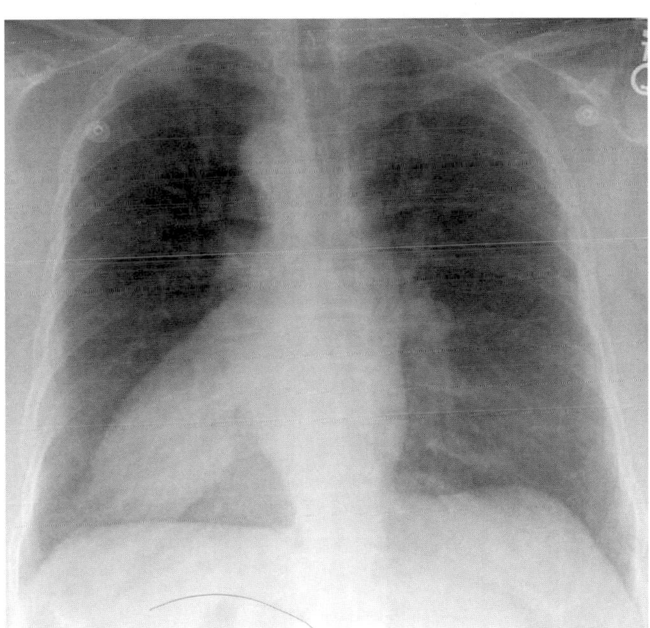

1. Where is the cardiac apex?
2. Where is the stomach bubble?
3. What is the diagnosis?
4. What is the incidence of congenital heart disease in this situation?

ANSWERS

CASE 60

Partial Anomalous Pulmonary Venous Connection

1. Partial anomalous pulmonary venous connection.
2. Left-to-right shunt.
3. Atrial level.
4. Sinus venosus atrial septal defect.

Reference

Reddy GP, Higgins CB. Magnetic resonance imaging of congenital heart disease: evaluation of morphology and function. *Semin Roentgenol* 38:342–351, 2003.

Cross-Reference

Cardiac Imaging: THE REQUISITES, 2nd edition, pp 320–323.

Comment

The MRI demonstrates a connection of the right upper lobe pulmonary vein to the superior vena cava. This is the most common type of partial anomalous pulmonary venous connection (PAPVC).

PAPVC is associated with other congenital abnormalities, most commonly a sinus venosus atrial septal defect, in which a connection exists between the left atrium and the superior vena cava as the cava enters the right atrium. Depending on the severity of the shunt, patients may be asymptomatic or may have dyspnea, cardiac murmur, and decreased exercise tolerance or may have pulmonary hypertension. Because it is an atrial-level shunt, PAPVC is physiologically similar to atrial septal defect.

Medical and surgical management depends on the accurate evaluation of the number and site of anomalous pulmonary veins and the presence of an atrial septal defect or other congenital anomaly. Gadolinium-enhanced MR angiography can accurately depict the presence, location, and size of anomalous veins in patients with PAPVC.

Notes

PAPVC - assc'd c̄ ASD
↳ Sinus venosus type

CASE 61

Situs Inversus with Dextrocardia

1. On the right.
2. On the right.
3. Situs inversus with dextrocardia.
4. Approximately 5% to 10%.

Reference

Spoon JM. Situs inversus totalis. *Neonatal Netw* 20:59–63, 2001.

Cross-Reference

Cardiac Imaging: THE REQUISITES, 2nd edition, pp 289–290.

Comment

The heart and stomach bubble are on the right, consistent with situs inversus with dextrocardia.

Most individuals who have situs inversus totalis can live into adulthood without intervention. There is an association with Kartagener (immotile cilia) syndrome, in which patients have bronchiectasis, sinusitis, and infertility. Only 5% to 10% of these individuals have a congenital cardiac lesion. On the other hand, situs ambiguus (visceral heterotaxy) or situs solitus with dextrocardia is strongly associated with complex congenital heart disease.

Imaging evaluation is usually straightforward: chest radiographs show that the cardiac apex is on the right, and the abdominal viscera are inverted. For a complete diagnosis, CT, MRI, or cineangiography can be used to identify the left-sided inferior vena cava entering the anatomic right atrium and the left-sided liver.

Notes

CASE 62

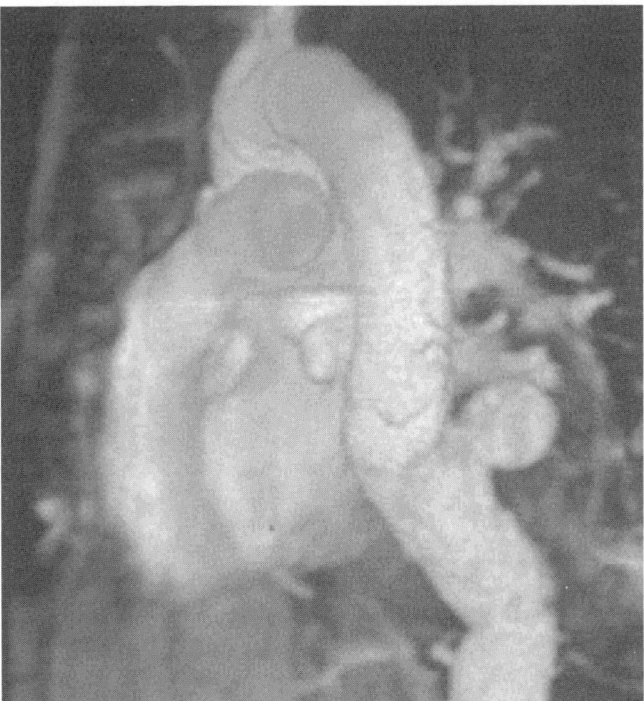

Volume-rendered gadolinium-enhanced MR angiogram

1. Which portion of the aorta is abnormal?
2. What is the diagnosis?
3. What are some possible etiologies?
4. What imaging modality is depicted?

CASE 62

Mycotic Pseudoaneurysm

1. Descending aorta.
2. Pseudoaneurysm.
3. Atherosclerosis (penetrating ulcer), mycotic infection, trauma, iatrogenic cause.
4. Volume-rendered image of a contrast-enhanced MR angiogram.

Reference

Gotway MB, Dawn SK. Thoracic aorta imaging with multislice CT. *Radiol Clin North Am* 41:521–543, 2003.

Cross-Reference

Cardiac Imaging: THE REQUISITES, 2nd edition, pp 388–392.

Comment

The MR angiogram shows an outpouching from the descending aorta. The neck of the outpouching is relatively narrow, suggestive of a pseudoaneurysm.

Etiologies of an aortic pseudoaneurysm include atherosclerosis (penetrating aortic ulcer), infection, trauma (deceleration injury—although this is an unusual location), and iatrogenic cause. In this patient, surgical pathology demonstrated a mycotic cause for the aneurysm. Pseudoaneurysms are characterized by disruption of one or more layers of the vessel wall, whereas true aneurysms have intact walls.

Evaluation is made by CT or MRI. Disruption of the wall is difficult to identify by imaging examination. However, many observers use a rule of thumb: a relatively narrow neck (less than 50% of the aneurysm diameter) suggests that the outpouching is a pseudoaneurysm, and a wide neck suggests a true aneurysm.

Notes

CASE 63

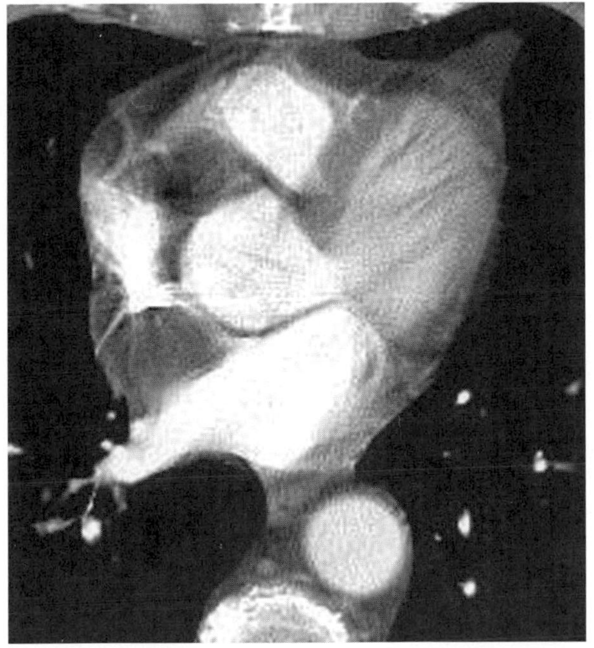
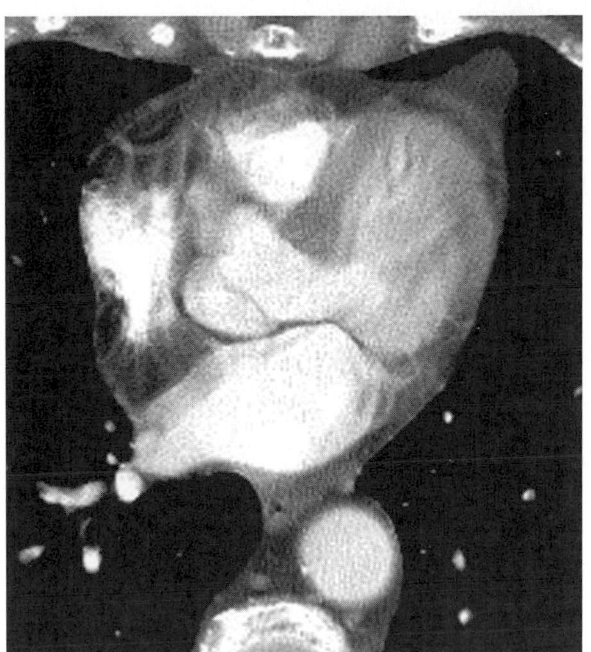

1. What is the density of the mass located between the left atrium and the uppermost portion of the right atrium?
2. What is the most likely diagnosis?
3. What symptom may be associated with this mass?
4. Does this lesion require surgery?

CASE 64

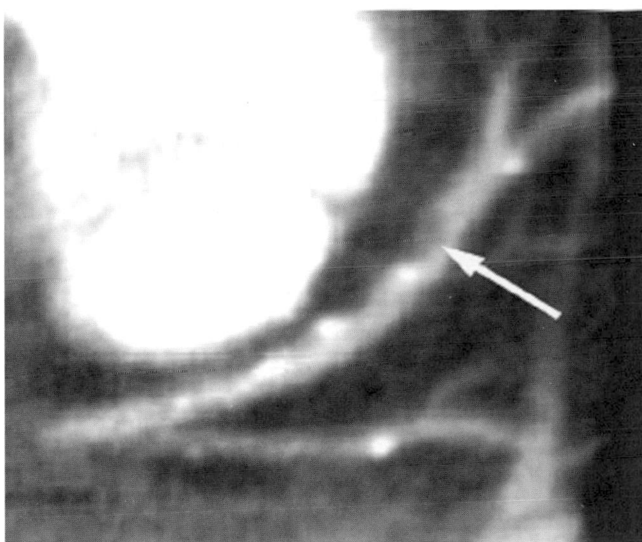

Multiplanar reformation of CT image.

1. What type of imaging examination is shown?
2. What is the diagnosis?
3. Is there calcification at the site of the lesion?
4. What would you suggest as the next step in diagnostic evaluation?

CASE 63

Lipomatous Hypertrophy of Interatrial Septum

1. Fat density.
2. Lipomatous hypertrophy of the interatrial septum.
3. Arrhythmia.
4. No.

Reference

Gaerte SC, Meyer CA, Winer-Muram HT, Tarver RD, Conces DJ, Jr. Fat-containing lesions of the chest. *Radiographics* 22(Special Issue):S61–S78, 2002.

Cross-Reference

Cardiac Imaging: THE REQUISITES, 2nd edition, pp 265–266.

Comment

There is a mass of fat density (approximately 30 Hounsfield units) between the right and left atria, consistent with lipomatous hypertrophy of the interatrial septum.

This lesion is benign and is characterized by fat in the interatrial septum. It occurs more frequently in elderly, obese patients and is associated with an increased amount of epicardial fat. Lipomatous hypertrophy of the interatrial septum can cause arrhythmia. It is important to recognize that the lesion is within the interatrial septum and to realize that it does not normally need to be resected.

The lesion is sometimes seen on echocardiography, and patients are referred to CT or MRI to differentiate intra-atrial lipoma or thrombus from lipomatous hypertrophy. In other instances, the mass is discovered incidentally on CT or MRI. When MRI is performed, fat saturation images can confirm the composition of the mass.

Notes

CASE 64

Coronary Artery Stenosis

1. Coronary CT angiography (CTA).
2. Stenosis of greater than 50% of the luminal diameter.
3. No; there is soft plaque *(arrow)*.
4. Stress perfusion scintigraphy. Alternatives are stress echocardiography, cardiac catheterization, and x-ray coronary angiography.

Reference

Schoepf UJ, Becker CR, Ohnesorge BM, Yucel EK. CT of coronary artery disease. *Radiology* 232:18–37, 2004.

Cross-Reference

Cardiac Imaging: THE REQUISITES, 2nd edition, pp 206–209.

Comment

The CT angiogram demonstrates marked stenosis of the left anterior descending coronary artery. There is no calcification at the site of narrowing, but there is an area of soft tissue density, suggestive of soft plaque.

Coronary CTA can be performed with electron-beam CT or with electrocardiographically gated multidetector helical CT. Promising results have come from studies using multidetector CT to identify coronary stenoses. CTA images can be reconstructed using a variety of methods, including curved multiplanar reformations and volume rendering.

The role of CTA is evolving in the diagnostic evaluation of patients with suspected or known coronary artery disease. Because of the high negative predictive value of CTA, patients with a normal CT coronary angiogram may not need further evaluation for coronary disease. On the other hand, patients with stenosis detected at CTA would need another study, such as stress perfusion scintigraphy, to confirm the significance of the lesion.

Notes

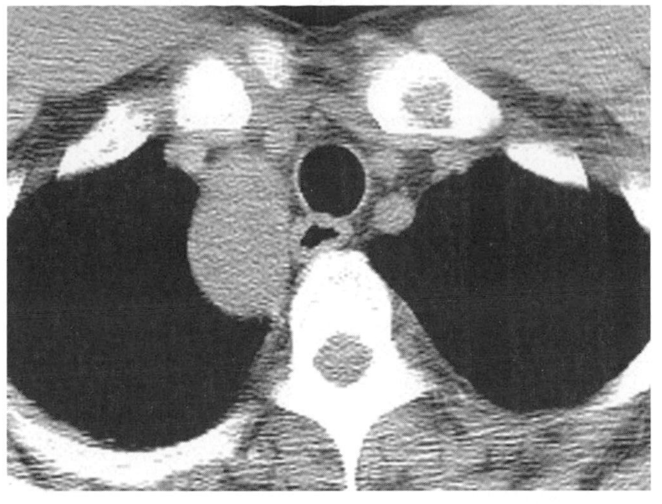
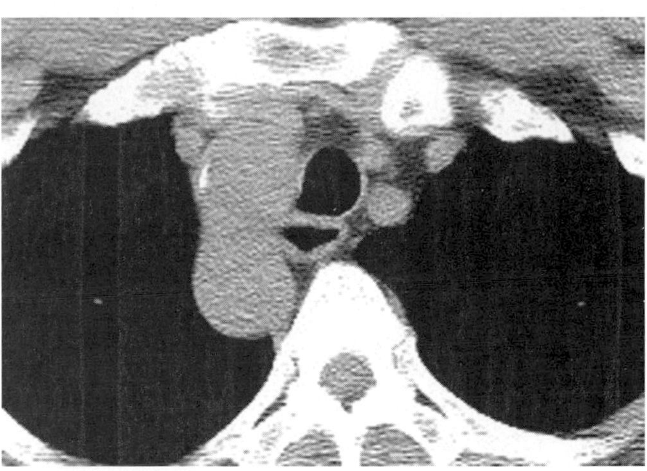
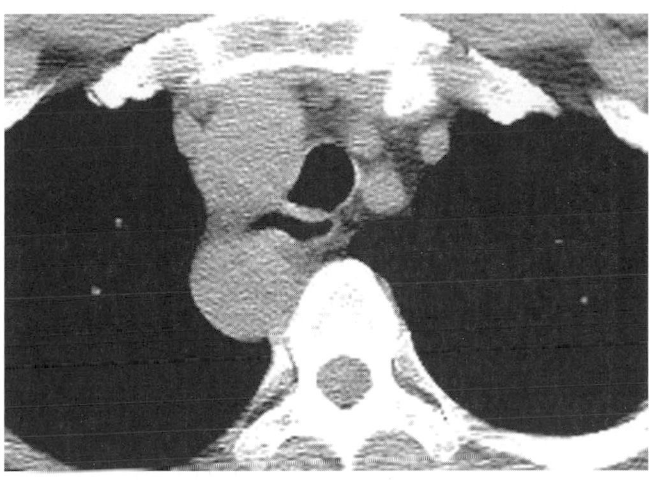
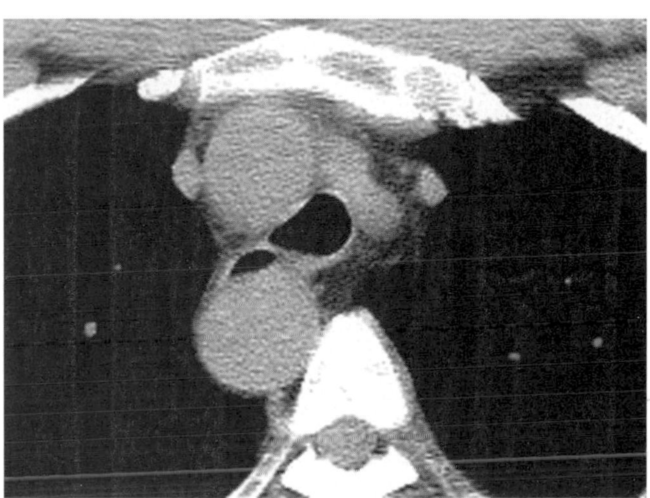

1. What is the arch anomaly?
2. Is this anomaly a vascular ring?
3. What is the incidence of associated congenital heart disease?
4. What congenital cardiac lesions are associated with this anomaly?

CASE 65

Mirror-Image Right Aortic Arch

1. Mirror-image right aortic arch.
2. No.
3. 95% to 98%.
4. Tetralogy of Fallot and truncus arteriosus.

Reference

Reddy GP, Higgins CB. Magnetic resonance imaging of congenital heart disease: evaluation of morphology and function. *Semin Roentgenol* 38:342–351, 2003.

Cross-Reference

Cardiac Imaging: THE REQUISITES, 2nd edition, p 407.

Comment

The unenhanced CT scan shows a right aortic arch. A left-sided brachiocephalic artery branches into the common carotid and subclavian arteries, and no aberrant vessel passes behind the esophagus.

Right aortic arch with mirror-image branching is not a vascular ring because no structure completes the ring posteriorly. More than 95% of individuals with a mirror-image right arch have cyanotic heart disease, most commonly tetralogy of Fallot or a variant. Truncus arteriosus is the second most common anomaly in these patients.

Imaging evaluation of arch anomalies usually consists of contrast-enhanced CT angiography or MR angiography. These studies delineate the vascular anatomy and document compression of the airway.

Notes

Asplenia =	(R) Isomerism	vs	Polysplenia (L) Isomerism
Bronchi	Epiarterial		Hyparterial
Minor Fissure	(B)		∅ minor
Heart	Cardiomegaly, complex CHD		Cardiomegaly, moderate CHD
Atrium	Common		ASD
Single Ventricle	~ 50%		DORV
Pulm Veins	TAPVC		PAPVC
Great Vessels	TGA (70%)		nl
SVC	(B) 50%		(B) ~ 30%
Bowel	Malrotation		malrotation
Clinically Age?	neonate		Infants
cyanosis	Yes		No
Issue	Infxn (asplenia)		None
Prognosis	Poor		Good
CHD	(L) TGA, pulm stenosis, single ventricle		PAPVC, ASD, VSD
Blood Smear	Heinz, Howell-Jolly Bodies		

CASE 66

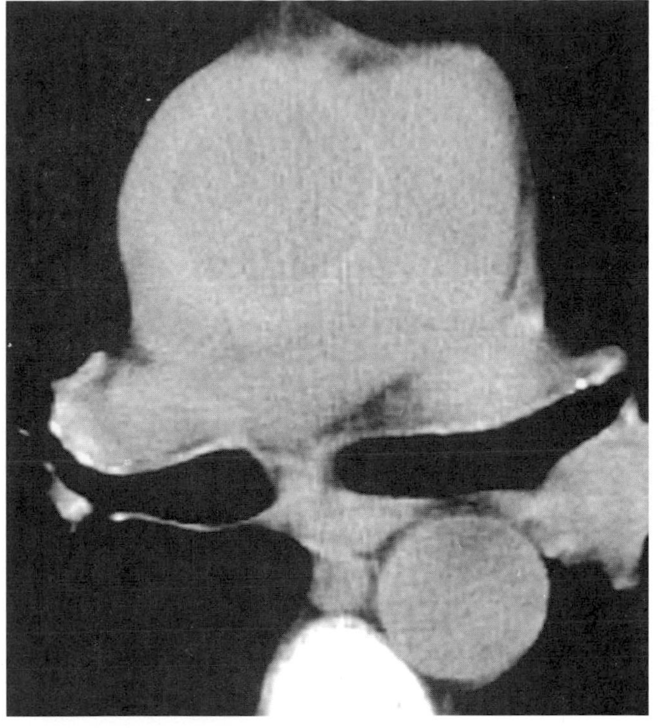

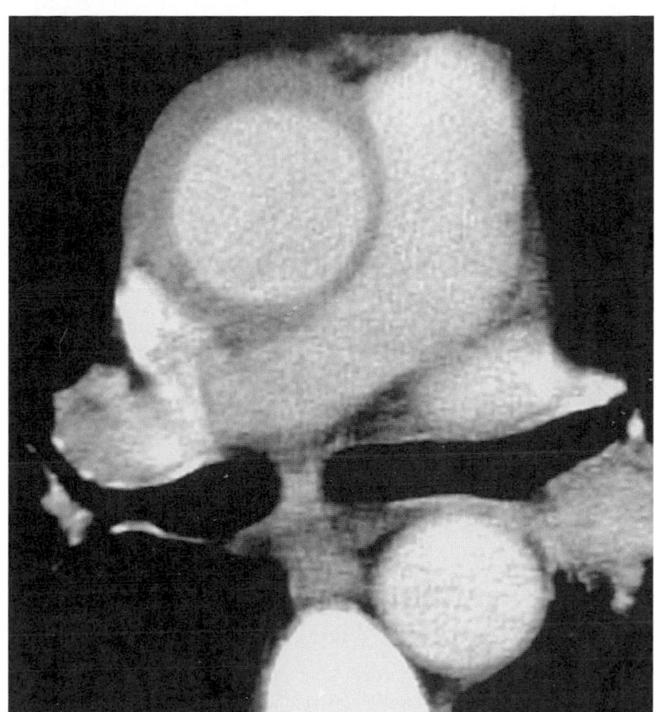

1. What are the abnormalities of the aorta?
2. What is the diagnosis?
3. What are vasa vasorum?
4. How does an intramural hematoma form?

CASE 67

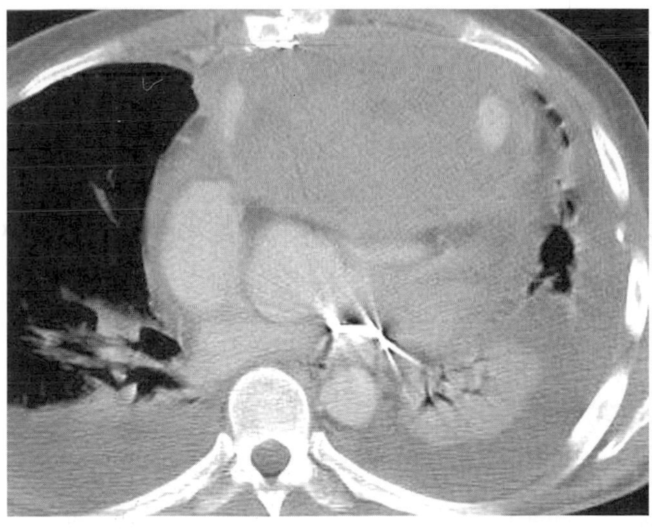

1. Where is the mass?
2. What is its density?
3. What is the most likely diagnosis?
4. Which cardiac chamber is most severely compressed?

CASE 66

Intramural Hematoma—Type A

1. Thickening of the wall of the ascending aorta. High density of the wall on the noncontrast image.
2. Stanford type A intramural hematoma.
3. Arteries that supply the walls of larger vessels, including the aorta.
4. Although there are various etiologies, most intramural hematomas develop as a result of vasa vasorum rupture in the aortic wall.

Reference

Gotway MB, Dawn SK. Thoracic aorta imaging with multislice CT. *Radiol Clin North Am* 41:521–543, 2003.

Cross-Reference

Cardiac Imaging: THE REQUISITES, 2nd edition, pp 402–406.

Comment

The wall of the ascending aorta is thickened. The noncontrast CT shows high density material in the aortic wall. These findings are consistent with an intramural hematoma.

An intramural hematoma most commonly develops as a result of vasa vasorum rupture in the aortic wall. Intramural hematoma is associated with systemic hypertension. The pathophysiology and natural history of an intramural hematoma are closely related to those of aortic dissection, and many authors think that intramural hematoma and dissection are different manifestations of the same disease. In other words, dissection begins as an intramural hematoma that eventually causes separation of the arterial wall and development of an intimal flap. Management of an intramural hematoma is usually similar to that of a frank dissection. Therefore, patients with Stanford type A dissection are usually treated surgically, whereas patients with a type B dissection can be managed medically.

Notes

CASE 67

Pericardial Hematoma

1. Pericardium.
2. Heterogeneous, with some high-attenuation areas.
3. Pericardial hematoma.
4. Right ventricle.

Reference

Wang ZJ, Reddy GP, Gotway MB, Yeh BM, Hetts SW, Higgins CB. CT and MR imaging of pericardial disease. *Radiographics* 23(Special Issue):S167–S180, 2003.

Cross-Reference

Cardiac Imaging: THE REQUISITES, 2nd edition, pp 256–258.

Comment

There is a large, heterogeneous mass anterior to the heart, separated from the cardiac chambers by a fat plane. The mass is most likely in the pericardium, but the image does not definitely establish the location in the pericardial space. The high-density areas are consistent with a hematoma. This patient was on a ventricular assist device and developed pericardial hemorrhage owing to a leak in the catheter system. The oval structures on either side of the hematoma are catheters.

A pericardial hematoma can result from trauma (iatrogenic or otherwise), myocardial infarction, aortic dissection, tumor, or pericarditis. When a hematoma is large enough to compress a cardiac chamber and cause hemodynamic compromise, it may have to be evacuated to relieve the compression.

On CT, a pericardial hematoma is characterized by high or heterogeneous density. A chronic hematoma can be calcified.

Notes

Pericardial Hematoma

DDx: - Trauma - incl iatrogenic

- MI
- Aortic Dissection
- Tumor
- Pericarditis

CASE 68

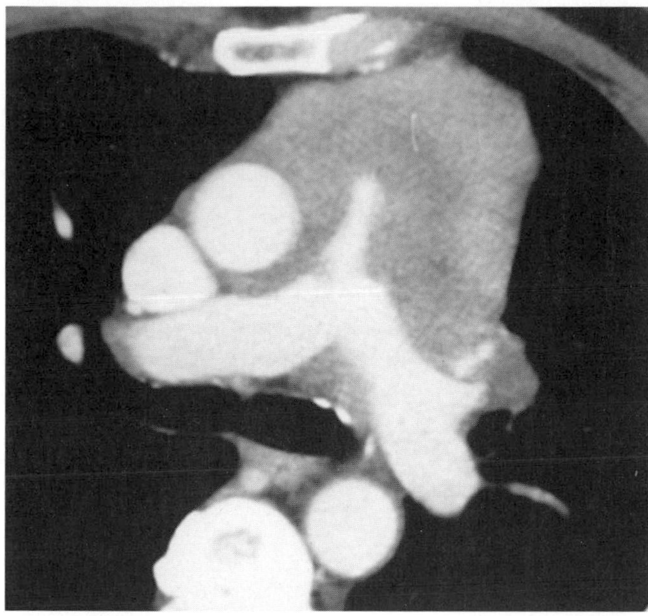

1. Where is the mass located?
2. What structures are compressed?
3. The noncontrast images demonstrated a homogeneous mass of soft tissue density. Is the mass a tumor or a hematoma?
4. Is the mass infiltrative?

ANSWERS

CASE 68

Pericardial Lymphoma

1. Pericardium.
2. Main pulmonary artery, proximal left pulmonary artery, and left superior pulmonary vein.
3. Tumor.
4. Yes.

Reference

Wang ZJ, Reddy GP, Gotway MB, Yeh BM, Hetts SW, Higgins CB. CT and MR imaging of pericardial disease. *Radiographics* 23(Special Issue):S167–S180, 2003.

Cross-Reference

Cardiac Imaging: THE REQUISITES, 2nd edition, p 261.

Comment

A large, heterogeneously enhancing mass is infiltrating the pericardium and compressing the pulmonary vessels. The enhancement excludes the diagnosis of hematoma. The infiltrative nature of the tumor suggests a malignant etiology. Biopsy yielded the diagnosis of lymphoma.

Most pericardial tumors are secondary to direct extension or metastasis from lung or breast carcinoma, lymphoma, and melanoma. Primary pericardial tumors are rare; mesothelioma is the most common. Primary pericardial lymphoma is associated with AIDS. Pleural effusion, including hemorrhagic effusion, occurs frequently. The prognosis of primary malignant pericardial tumors is poor.

CT is frequently performed for diagnosis, but MRI is especially useful to define the extent of involvement.

Notes

Pericardial Tumor
DDx - · Met / Ext from Lung, Breast Ca
· Melanoma
- 1° Mesothelioma
- Lymphoma

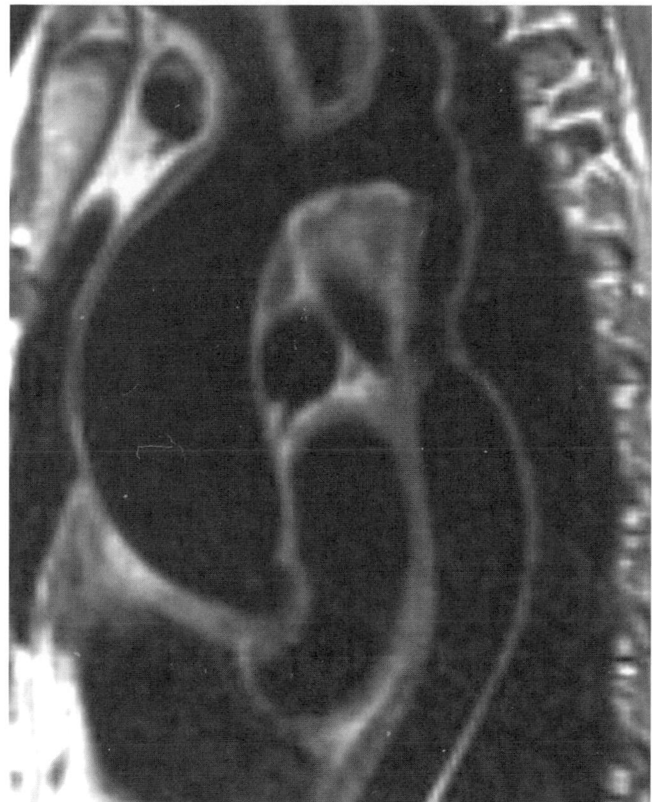

Oblique sagittal spin-echo MR image.

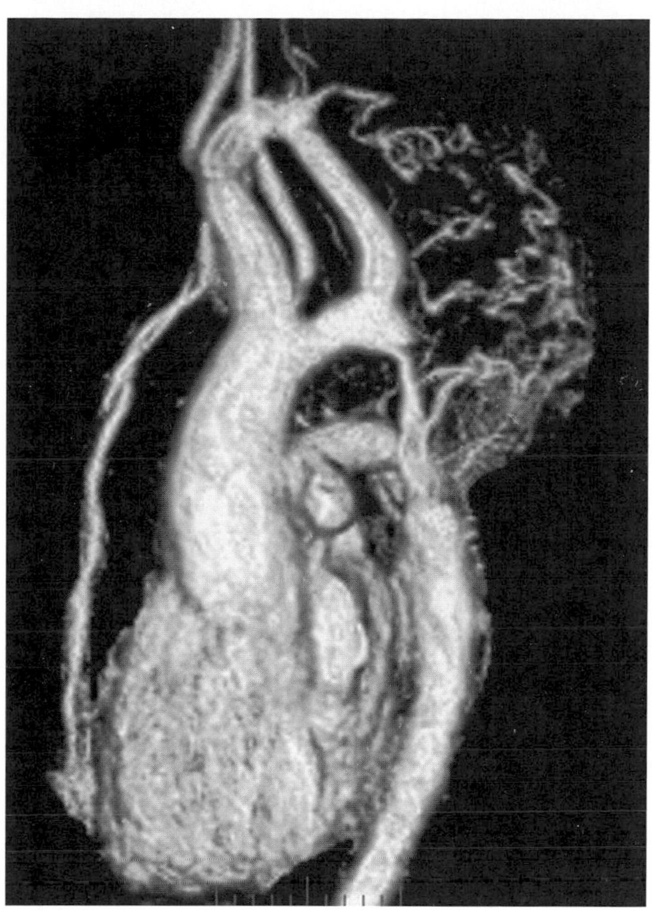

Volume-rendered gadolinium-enhanced MR angiogram.

1. Which portion of the aorta is narrowed?
2. Are collateral vessels present?
3. What is the most common form of coarctation?
4. What are some acquired causes of coarctation?

ANSWERS

CASE 69

Takayasu Arteritis—Long-Segment Coarctation of Aorta

1. Proximal descending aorta.
2. Yes.
3. Discrete, juxtaductal coarctation.
4. Takayasu arteritis, giant cell arteritis (rare).

Reference

Gotway MB, Araoz PA, Macedo TA, et al. Imaging findings in Takayasu's arteritis. *AJR Am J Roentgenol* 184:1945–1950, 2005.

Cross-Reference

Cardiac Imaging: THE REQUISITES, 2nd edition, pp 384–387.

Comment

The MR images demonstrate a long-segment stenosis of the proximal descending aorta. The contrast-enhanced MR angiogram shows large collateral vessels. The patient carried a diagnosis of Takayasu arteritis, which is a cause of aortic narrowing.

Congenital coarctation is most commonly discrete and juxtaductal in location. Long-segment coarctations may be acquired; Takayasu arteritis is an important cause. Takayasu arteritis can also cause narrowing of the arch vessels and of the abdominal aorta and its branches. Takayasu arteritis most commonly is diagnosed in young women. Patients typically have nonspecific systemic symptoms during the active phase of the disease. In the sclerotic phase, symptoms of vascular insufficiency develop: abdominal angina and claudication. Hypertension is frequent.

On MRI, the active phase of the disease manifests as wall thickening and enhancement. In the sclerotic phase, MR angiography can demonstrate areas of stenosis.

Notes

Acquired Coarctation DDx. - Takayasu Arteritis
- Giant Cell Arteritis

CASE 70

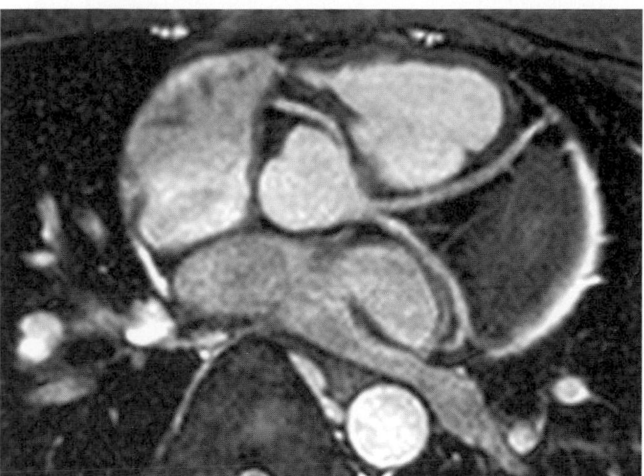

Reconstruction of coronary MR angiogram.

1. What type of study does the figure represent?
2. Which vessel is anomalous?
3. What is the course of the anomalous vessel?
4. Does this anomaly require treatment?

CASE 70

Anomalous Right Coronary Artery

1. MRI (coronary MR angiogram).
2. Right coronary artery.
3. Interarterial: between the aorta and pulmonary outflow tract.
4. Yes; reimplantation or bypass surgery.

Reference

Danias PG, Stuber M, McConnell MV, Manning WJ. The diagnosis of congenital coronary anomalies with magnetic resonance imaging. *Coron Artery Dis* 12:621–626, 2001.

Cross-Reference

Cardiac Imaging: THE REQUISITES, 2nd edition, pp 223–225.

Comment

The coronary MR angiogram shows anomalous origin of the right coronary artery from the left coronary cusp. The anomalous vessel passes in an interarterial course between the aortic root and the pulmonary outflow tract.

There are several types of coronary artery anomalies. The interarterial course is thought to predispose the artery to compression and cause ischemia, leading to angina, arrhythmia, syncope, or sudden death (cardiac arrest). Most cardiac surgeons would recommend reimplantation of the anomalous artery or bypass surgery. On the other hand, if the anomalous artery passes posterior to the aorta, the artery does not become compressed, and surgery is not necessary.

X-ray coronary angiography can demonstrate a coronary anomaly but might not be able to show the course of the vessel. Therefore, MR angiography and electrocardiographically gated CT are the preferred methods for identification of the arterial course.

Notes

Coronary Anomalies 1) Interarterial

(R) Coronary 2) Posterior

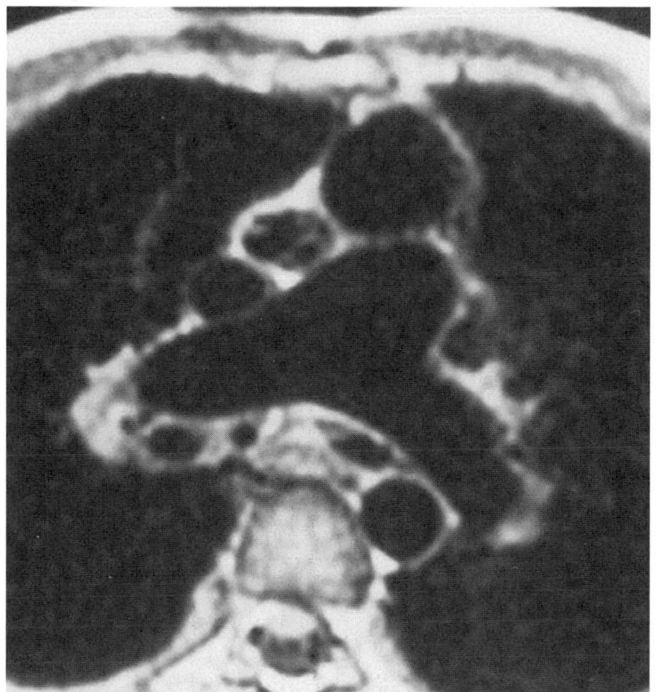

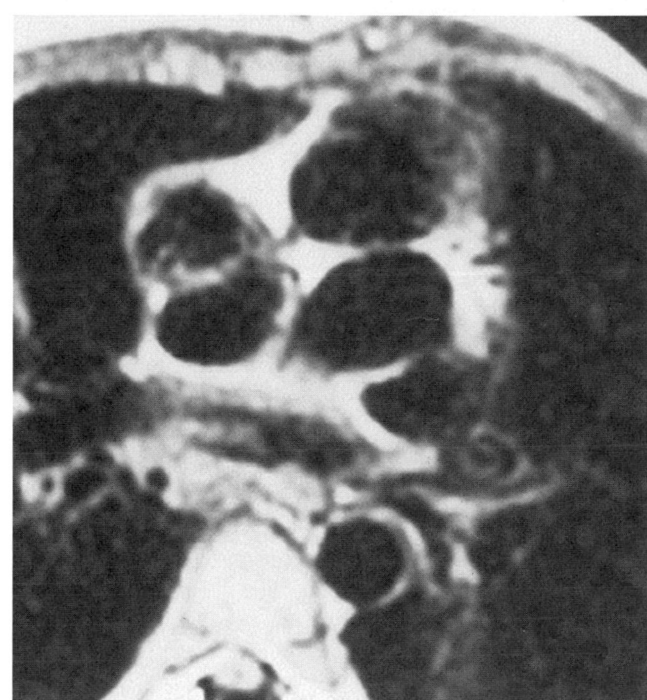

Axial spin-echo MR images.

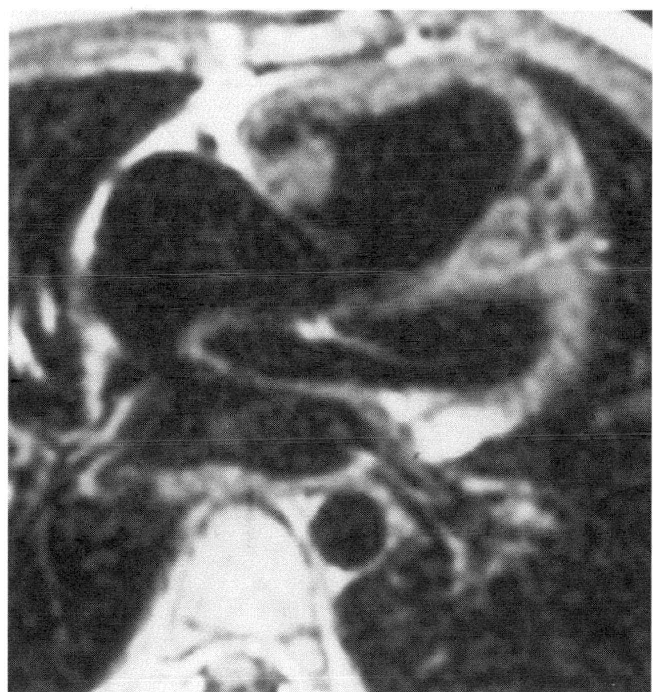

1. What is the relationship of the ascending aorta to the main pulmonary artery?
2. Which ventricle gives rise to the aorta?
3. Which ventricle gives rise to the pulmonary artery?
4. What is the diagnosis?

CASE 71

Complete Transposition of the Great Arteries

1. The aorta is anterior to the pulmonary artery.
2. The right ventricle.
3. The left ventricle.
4. Transposition of the great arteries.

Reference

Reddy GP, Higgins CB. Magnetic resonance imaging of congenital heart disease: evaluation of morphology and function. *Semin Roentgenol* 38:342–351, 2003.

Cross-Reference

Cardiac Imaging: THE REQUISITES, 2nd edition, pp 303–305.

Comment

The MR image shows that the ascending aorta is anterior to the main pulmonary artery. The right ventricle gives rise to the aorta, and the left ventricle to the pulmonary artery, consistent with transposition of the great arteries. The right ventricle is hypertrophied and enlarged. The patient has undergone a Senning procedure with an atrial baffle.

Transposition of the great arteries is an admixture lesion with resultant shunt vascularity and cyanosis. Patients have an intracardiac shunt such as a ventricular or atrial septal defect. Operative repair involves an arterial switch, or Jatene, procedure. In the past, patients underwent a Mustard or Senning procedure with an atrial baffle.

MRI is used primarily to assess postoperative function, especially that of the right ventricle, and to detect postoperative complications such as baffle thrombosis or pulmonary artery stenosis after an arterial switch procedure.

Notes

CASE 72

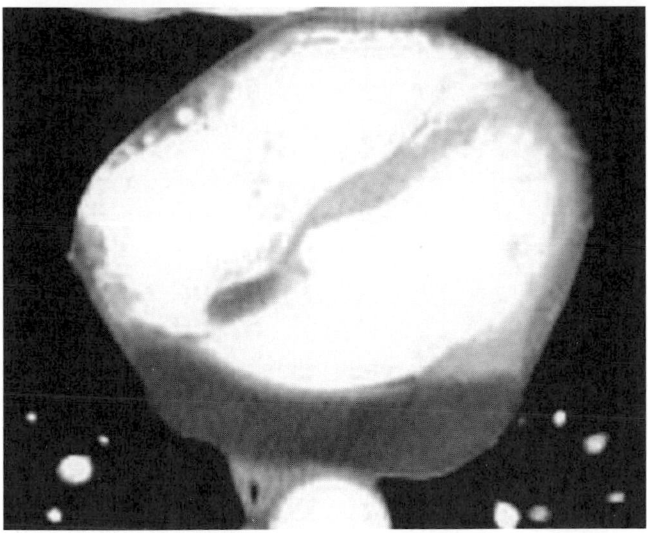

1. What is the density of the mass?
2. Where is the mass located?
3. Is the mass compressing the cardiac chambers?
4. What is the most likely diagnosis?

CASE 73

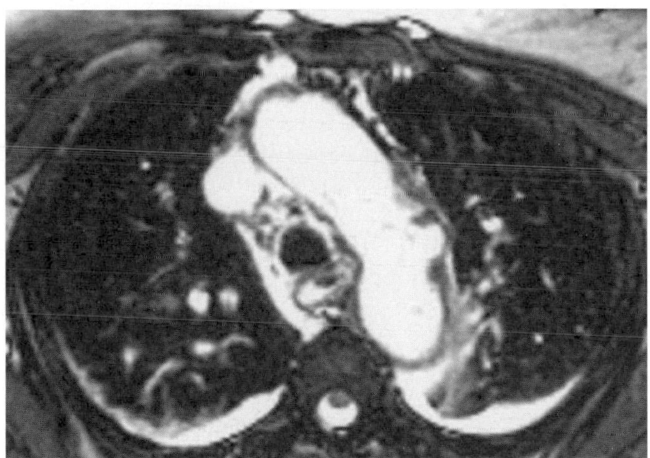

Axial gradient-echo cine-MR image.

1. What are some causes of acute aortic syndrome?
2. What is the etiology of a penetrating aortic ulcer?
3. What are the complications of a penetrating aortic ulcer?
4. What is the management of a penetrating aortic ulcer?

CASE 72

Pericardial Lipoma

1. It is of low density.
2. In the pericardium.
3. No.
4. Pericardial lipoma.

Reference

Wang ZJ, Reddy GP, Gotway MB, Yeh BM, Hetts SW, Higgins CB. CT and MR imaging of pericardial disease. *Radiographics* 23(Special Issue):S167–S180, 2003.

Cross-Reference

Cardiac Imaging: THE REQUISITES, 2nd edition, pp 265–266.

Comment

The CT scan reveals a homogeneous, low-density mass in the pericardium, consistent with a lipoma.

Cardiac lipoma most commonly occurs in the right atrium. Pericardial lipoma is less common. Lipomas tend to be soft and flexible, and even large tumors may not compress the heart. Fat-saturation MRI sequences are ideal for demonstrating that the mass is composed of fat.

Notes

CASE 73

Penetrating Aortic Ulcer

1. Aortic dissection, ruptured/leaking aneurysm, and penetrating aortic ulcer.
2. Atherosclerosis with plaque ulceration.
3. Aortic rupture/leak and pseudoaneurysm formation.
4. Ascending aorta: may require surgery. Descending aorta: managed medically.

Reference

Gotway MB, Dawn SK. Thoracic aorta imaging with multislice CT. *Radiol Clin North Am* 41:521–543, 2003.

Cross-Reference

Cardiac Imaging: THE REQUISITES, 2nd edition, pp 402–403.

Comment

The contrast-enhanced CT scan demonstrates atherosclerosis in the aortic arch. At the lateral aspect of the arch, there is an area of hypoattenuation, consistent with plaque. There is ulceration of the plaque and the ulcer extends outside the confines of the aortic wall, indicating that it is a penetrating ulcer.

When plaque ulcerates, disrupts the intima, and extends into the media, the process is termed a penetrating aortic ulcer. A penetrating ulcer can form a pseudoaneurysm. If the ulcer extends through the aortic wall, aortic rupture or leak can occur. The most common location is the mid-descending aorta. If a penetrating ulcer is located in the ascending aorta, it is usually repaired surgically. Descending aortic penetrating ulcers can be managed medically.

CT and MRI can both demonstrate the ulcer, as well as associated intramural hematoma or aortic rupture.

Notes

CASE 74

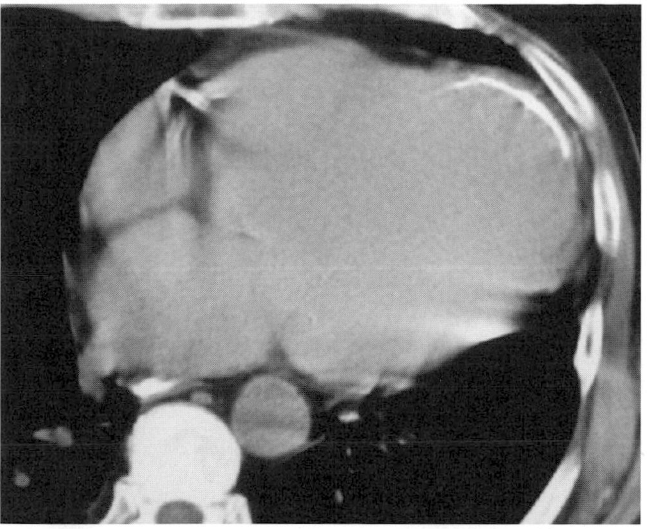

1. Where is the calcification?
2. What is the differential diagnosis?
3. What findings on MRI would confirm an aneurysm?
4. What is the indication for surgery?

CASE 75

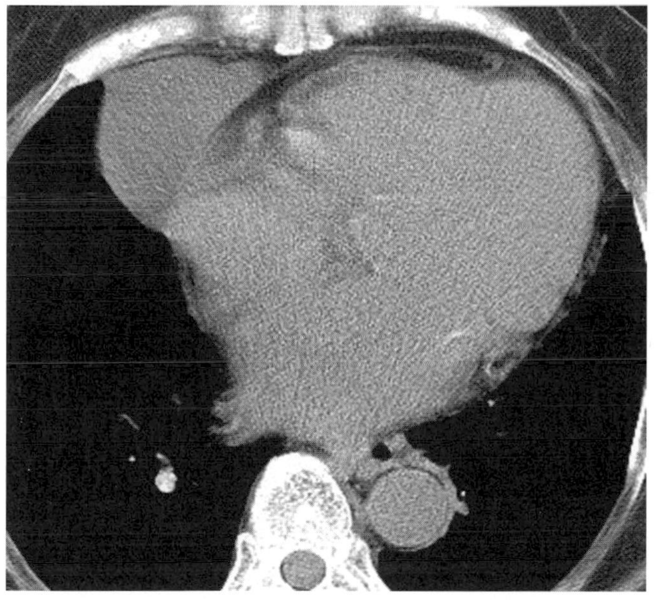

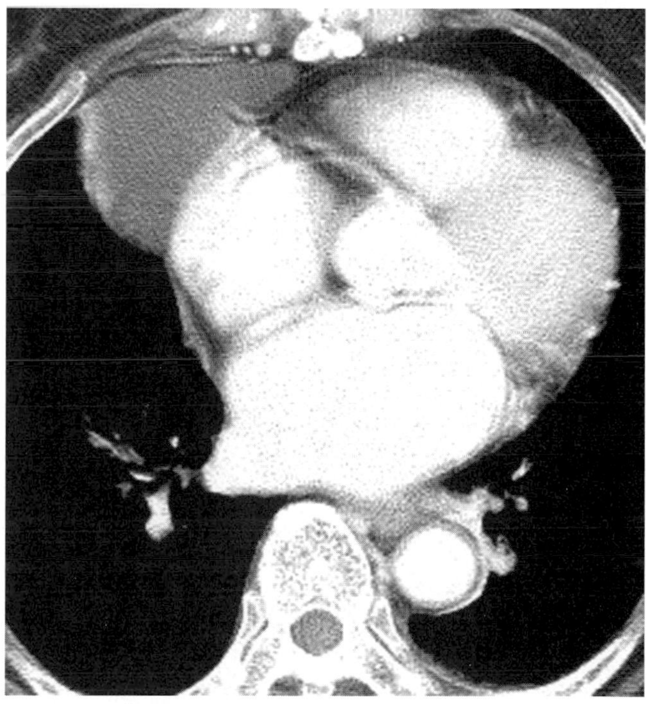

1. Where is the mass?
2. Is it well-circumscribed?
3. Is the mass malignant or benign?
4. If the density of the mass is 35 Hounsfield units on the noncontrast image and 36 Hounsfield units on the contrast-enhanced image, what is the most likely diagnosis?

CASE 74

Calcified Left Ventricular Aneurysm

1. Left ventricular apex.
2. Calcified left ventricular aneurysm, calcified infarct, calcified thrombus.
3. Paradoxical motion during systole.
4. To improve clinical function.

Reference

White RD. MR and CT assessment for ischemic cardiac disease. *J Magn Reson Imaging* 19:659–675, 2004.

Cross-Reference

Cardiac Imaging: THE REQUISITES, 2nd edition, pp 234–241.

Comment

The calcification in the apex of the left ventricle can reflect an aneurysm, prior myocardial infarction, or calcification of a thrombus. Thrombi are usually oval or round, rather than linear. The prominence of the apex suggests a true aneurysm. This can be confirmed by the observation of paradoxical motion on echocardiography, cine-MRI, cine-CT, or ventriculography. Because true aneurysms are not at risk for rupture, aneurysmectomy is not required but can be performed to improve function.

Transmural myocardial infarction is the cause of left ventricular aneurysms. True aneurysms typically are located in the anteroapical region of the left ventricle and have wide necks.

Notes

Location of True Aneurysms = Antero-Apical

- DDx
  - Calcified LV Aneurysm
  - Calcified infarct
  - Calcified thrombus

CASE 75

Pericardial Cyst

1. Right cardiophrenic sulcus.
2. Yes.
3. Benign.
4. Pericardial cyst.

Reference

Wang ZJ, Reddy GP, Gotway MB, Yeh BM, Hetts SW, Higgins CB. CT and MR imaging of pericardial disease. *Radiographics* 23(Special Issue):S167–S180, 2003.

Cross-Reference

Cardiac Imaging: THE REQUISITES, 2nd edition, pp 256–258.

Comment

The CT scan demonstrates a well-circumscribed, homogeneous mass that does not enhance. The mass has no malignant features. The lack of enhancement and location adjacent to the pericardium suggest that it is a pericardial cyst.

Pericardial cysts are usually homogeneous and well circumscribed. Often they contain simple fluid, but they can contain complex fluid that produces higher attenuation on CT, as in this case. The diagnosis can be confirmed by the lack of enhancement on CT or MRI or uniform high signal intensity on T2-weighted MRI.

Notes

CASE 78

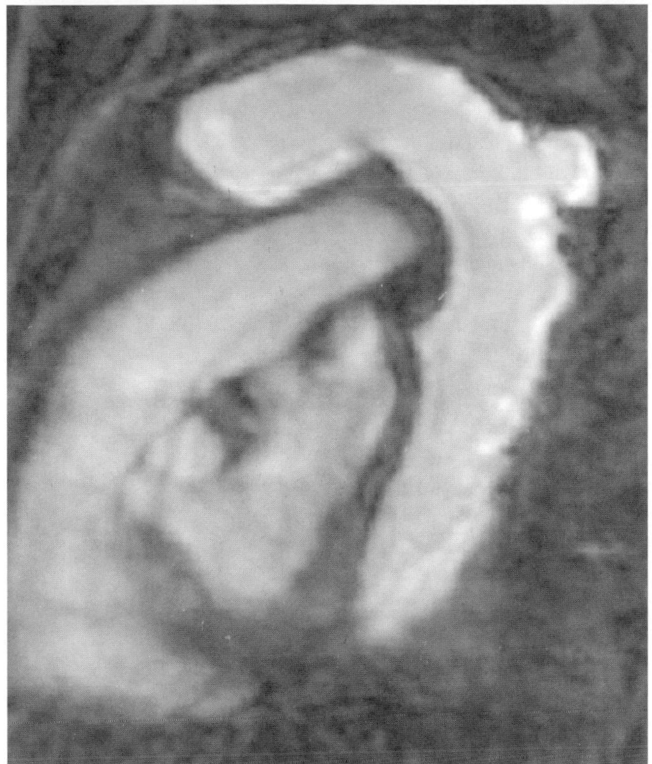

Gadolinium-enhanced MR angiogram.

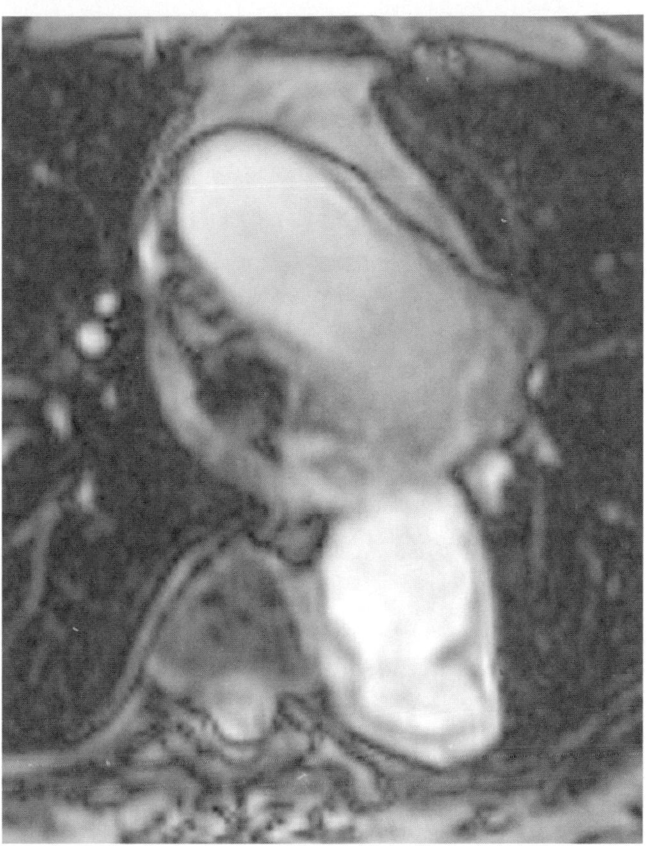

Axial gradient-echo cine-MR image.

1. Is this a pseudoaneurysm or a true aneurysm?
2. What are some possible causes of this finding?
3. What is the most appropriate management?
4. What imaging sequences are shown?

ANSWERS

CASE 78

Pseudoaneurysm Secondary to Penetrating Ulcer

1. Pseudoaneurysm.
2. Atherosclerosis (penetrating ulcer), mycotic infection, trauma, iatrogenic cause.
3. Surgical resection.
4. Sagittal section of a contrast-enhanced MR angiogram and axial cine-MRI.

Reference

Reddy GP, Higgins CB. MR imaging of the thoracic aorta. *Magn Reson Imaging Clin N Am* 8:1–15, 2000.

Cross-Reference

Cardiac Imaging: THE REQUISITES, 2nd edition, pp 402–403.

Comment

The MR angiogram shows an outpouching from the distal arch. The neck of the aneurysm is relatively narrow, suggestive of a pseudoaneurysm. An aortic pseudoaneurysm can be due to a penetrating atherosclerotic ulcer, infection, trauma (deceleration injury—although this is an unusual location), or iatrogenic injury. In this patient, the presence of extensive atherosclerosis in the aorta suggests that the etiology is a penetrating ulcer.

Because pseudoaneurysms are characterized by disruption of one or more layers of the arterial wall, they are at risk for rupture, and management usually involves surgical resection.

CT or MRI can be used to establish the diagnosis. If the outpouching has a relatively narrow neck (less than 50% of the aneurysm diameter), it is likely a pseudoaneurysm, whereas an aneurysm with a wide neck is likely to be a true aneurysm.

Notes

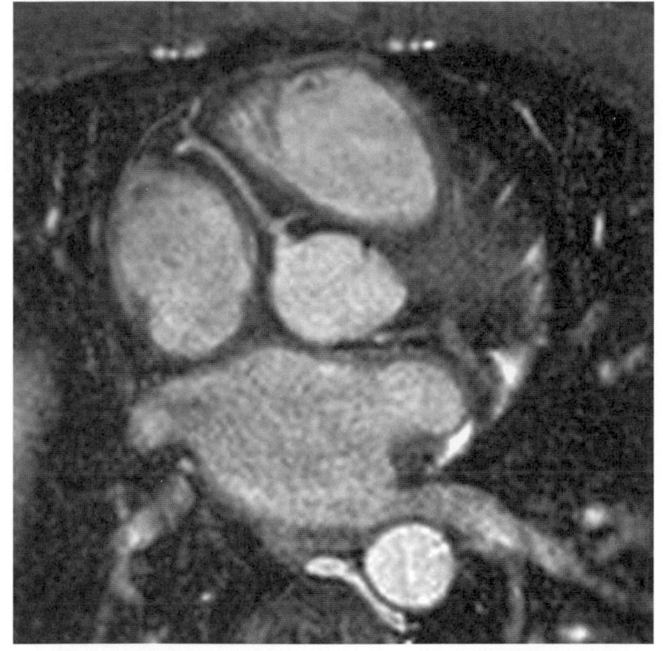

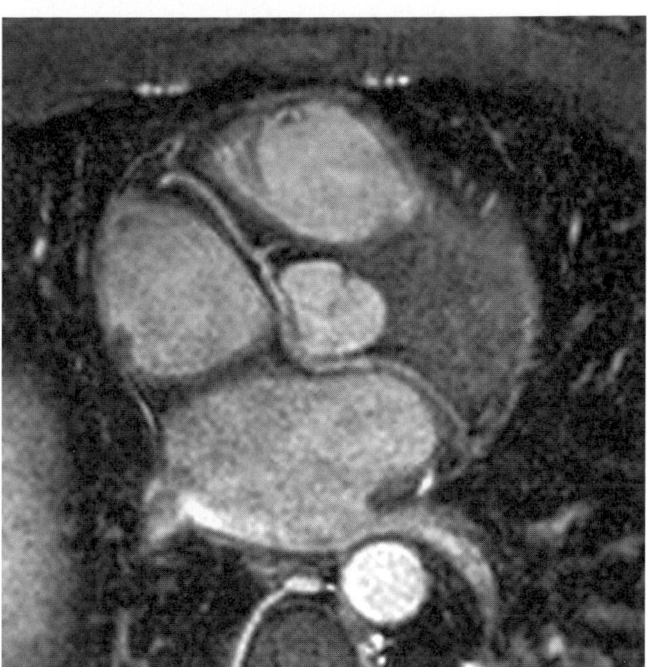

"Soap-bubble" reconstruction of coronary MR angiogram.

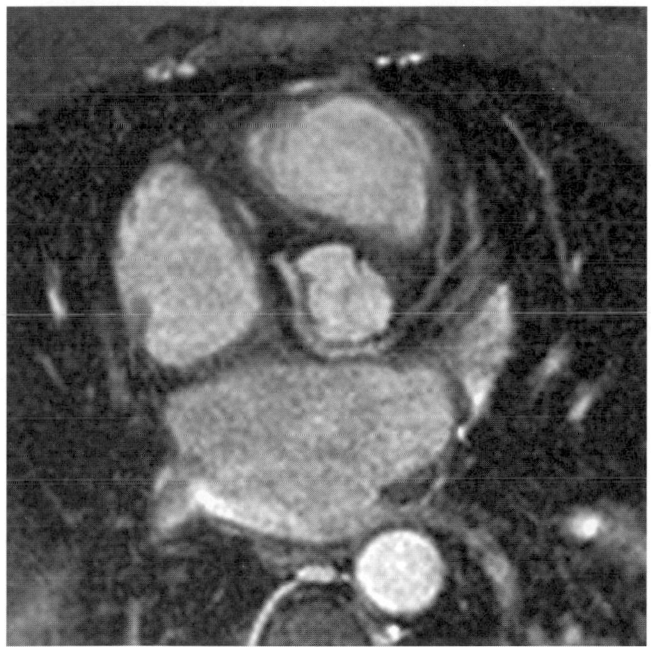

1. Which coronary artery is anomalous?
2. Is there a common origin of the right and left coronary arteries?
3. What is the course of the anomalous vessel?
4. Does this anomaly require treatment?

CASE 79

Anomalous Left Coronary Artery

1. Left main coronary artery.
2. Yes.
3. Retroaortic.
4. No.

Reference

Danias PG, Stuber M, McConnell MV, Manning WJ. The diagnosis of congenital coronary anomalies with magnetic resonance imaging. *Coron Artery Dis* 12:621–626, 2001.

Cross-Reference

Cardiac Imaging: THE REQUISITES, 2nd edition, pp 223–225.

Comment

The navigator-gated coronary MR angiogram demonstrates an anomalous origin of the left main coronary artery from the right coronary artery. An anomalous coronary artery usually arises directly from the aorta, and this common origin ("single coronary artery") is rare. The anomalous left coronary artery passes posterior to the ascending aorta and gives rise to the left anterior descending and left circumflex arteries.

There are several types of coronary artery anomaly. The interarterial course can subject the artery to compression and cause ischemia, with possible angina, arrhythmia, syncope, or sudden death, suggesting the need for surgical correction. In contrast, an anomalous course posterior to the aorta will not cause symptoms; it is considered to be a normal variant that does not need treatment.

X-ray coronary angiography can detect a coronary anomaly but often cannot definitively identify the course of the vessel. Therefore, MR angiography and electrocardiographically gated CT are used to map the course of the anomalous vessel.

Notes

Challenge

CASE 80

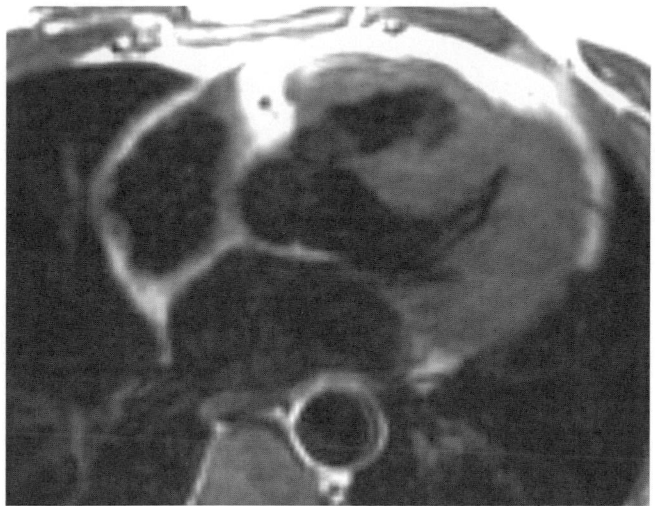

Axial spin-echo cine-MR image.

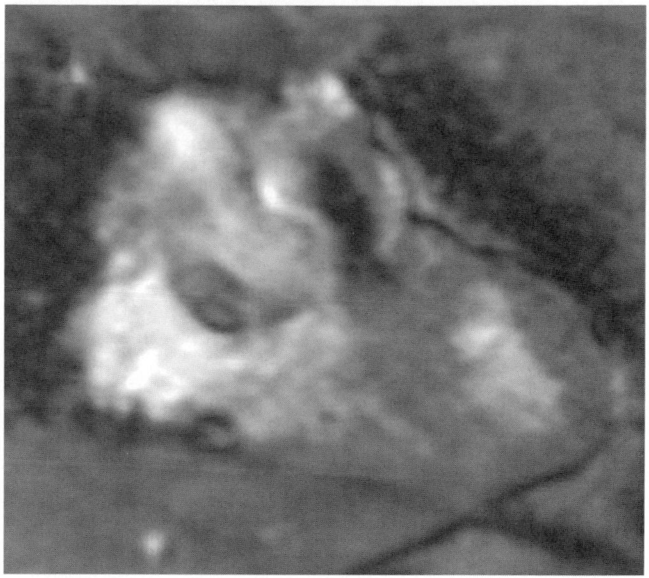

Coronal gradient-echo cine-MR image.

1. What type of ventricular septal defect is present?
2. What is the role of MRI in the evaluation of this type of defect?
3. On the cine-MR image, what does the black jet in the pulmonary artery indicate?
4. What are some complications of this lesion?

CASE 80

Supracristal Ventricular Septal Defect

1. A supracristal ventricular septal defect.
2. The lesion has a characteristic appearance on axial MRI, with a defect between the base of the aorta and the right ventricular infundibulum. It may be difficult to evaluate the lesion with echocardiography.
3. A left-to-right shunt.
4. Aortic insufficiency, or sinus of Valsalva prolapse or aneurysm.

Reference

Bremerich J, Reddy GP, Higgins CB. MRI of supracristal ventricular septal defects. *J Comput Assist Tomogr* 23:13–15, 1999.

Cross-Reference

Cardiac Imaging: THE REQUISITES, 2nd edition, pp 331–334.

Comment

The axial spin-echo image demonstrates a defect between the base of the aorta and the right ventricular outflow tract, consistent with a supracristal ventricular septal defect. The coronal cine image shows a black flow jet propagating into the pulmonary artery, consistent with a left-to-right shunt.

A supracristal ventricular septal defect is also known as doubly committed subarterial defect because its location is both subaortic and subpulmonary.

Echocardiography is the primary imaging modality for the evaluation of intracardiac shunts. However, because of the location of a supracristal ventricular septal defect, it may be difficult to assess with echocardiography. MRI demonstrates the characteristic appearance of a connection between the aortic root and right ventricular outflow tract.

Notes

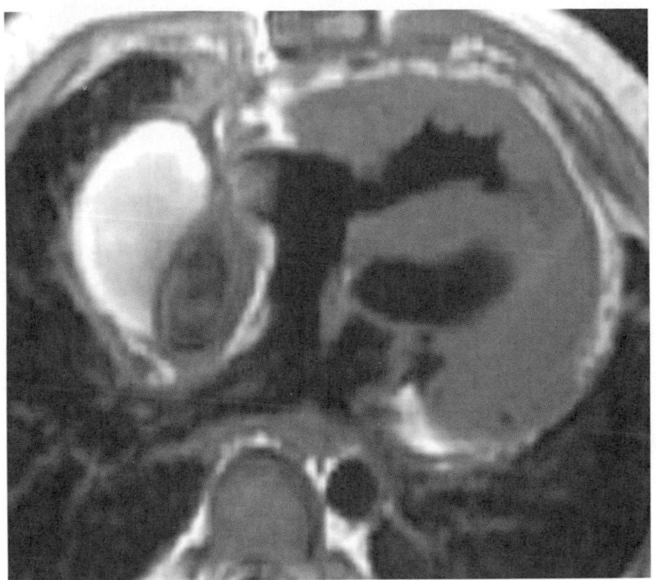

Axial spin-echo MR image.

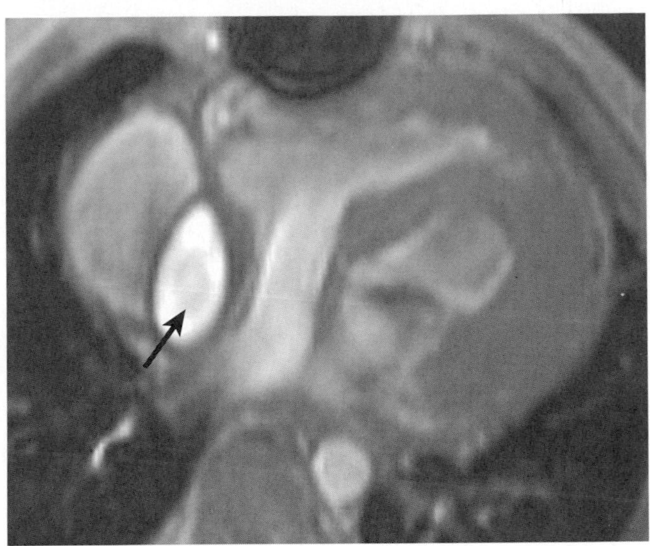

Axial gradient-echo cine-MR image.

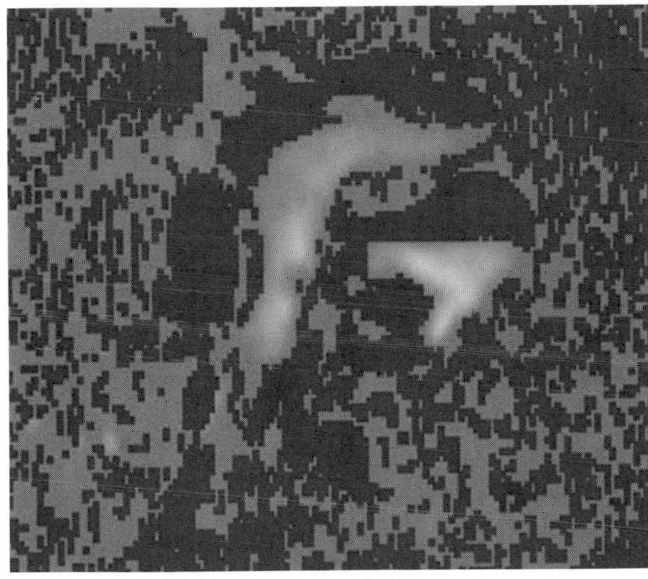

Velocity-encoded cine-MR phase-contrast image.

1. What is a Fontan shunt?
2. What lesions can be treated with a Fontan procedure?
3. Is the Fontan shunt *(arrow)* patent?
4. What is the high-signal-intensity structure to the right of the Fontan shunt?

CASE 81

Hypoplastic Left Heart Syndrome—Postoperative with Fontan Shunt

1. A shunt between the inferior vena cava and the pulmonary artery, bypassing the heart.
2. Tricuspid atresia, hypoplastic left heart syndrome (as part of the Norwood procedure).
3. Yes.
4. A hematoma.

Reference

Bardo DM, Frankel DG, Applegate KE, Murphy DJ, Saneto RP. Hypoplastic left heart syndrome. *Radiographics* 21:705–717, 2001.

Cross-Reference

Cardiac Imaging: THE REQUISITES, 2nd edition, pp 355–359.

Comment

MRI was performed to assess the patency of the Fontan shunt in a patient with hypoplastic left heart syndrome. On the spin-echo image, intermediate signal intensity in the shunt may indicate slow flow or a thrombus. The cine-MR image shows uniform high signal, consistent with patency and lack of thrombus. The mass to the right of the Fontan shunt has high signal intensity on the spin-echo and gradient-echo cine images. The velocity-encoded cine phase-contrast image demonstrates the lack of flow in the mass. These findings are consistent with a postoperative hematoma.

Notes

CASE 82

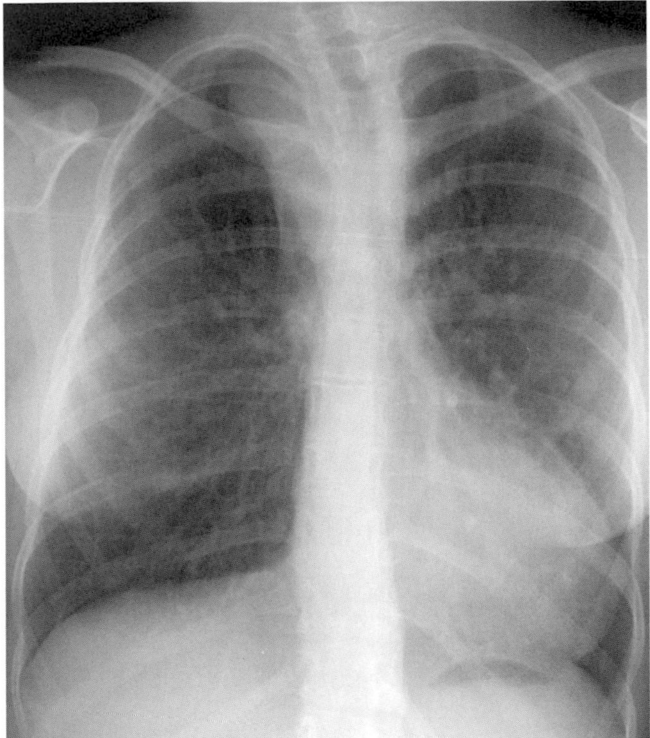

1. What is the differential diagnosis?
2. Is a biopsy of the mass appropriate?
3. On which side is the aortic arch?
4. Which primitive arch forms the normal aortic arch?

CASE 82

Cervical Aortic Arch

1. Aneurysm of aortic arch, aneurysm of right subclavian or common carotid arteries, cervical aortic arch, lymphadenopathy.
2. No!
3. Right.
4. The left fourth arch.

References

McElhinney DB, Tworetzky W, Hanley FL, Rudolph AM. Congenital obstructive lesions of the right aortic arch. *Ann Thorac Surg* 67:1194–1202, 1999.

Hirao K, Miyazaki A, Noguchi M, Shibata R, Hayashi K. The cervical aortic arch with aneurysm formation. *J Comput Assist Tomogr* 23:959–962, 1999.

Comment

The chest radiograph shows a mass in the right side of the superior mediastinum. The aortic arch is on the right side. By history, the patient had a pulsatile mass in the right supraclavicular region. Further imaging showed it to be a cervical aortic arch.

Cervical aortic arch is a rare anomaly in which the arch arises from the primitive third arch instead of the fourth. It may be more common on the right side. It has been reported that the ipsilateral internal and external carotid and the vertebral arteries arise directly from the arch. Cervical aortic arch is usually asymptomatic but can present as a pulsatile mass in the supraclavicular fossa or neck, with obstruction due to kinking, or as an aneurysm.

Diagnosis is based on the presence of the aortic arch near the base of the neck. Some authors state that the diagnosis depends on the finding of separate origins of the internal and external carotid arteries directly from the arch.

Notes

CASE 83

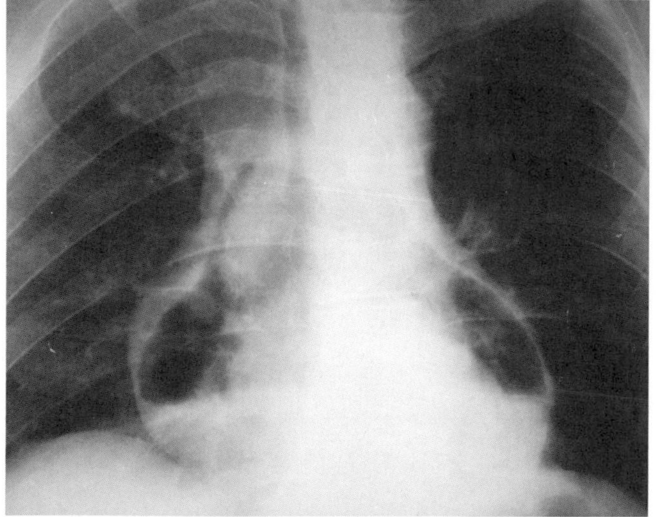

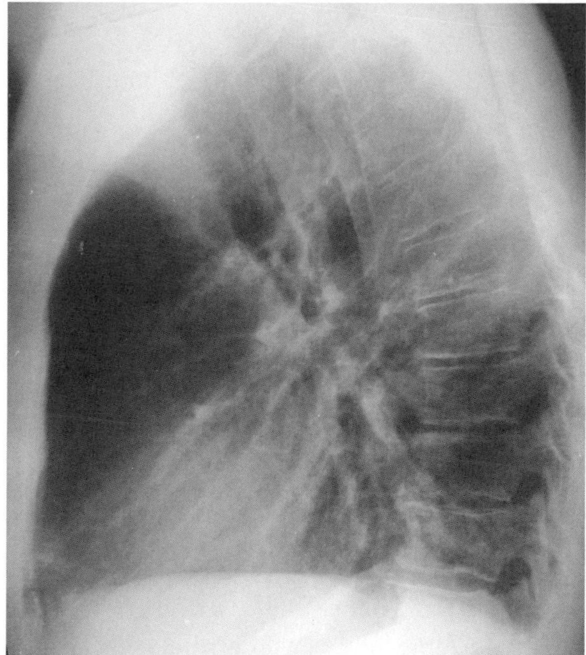

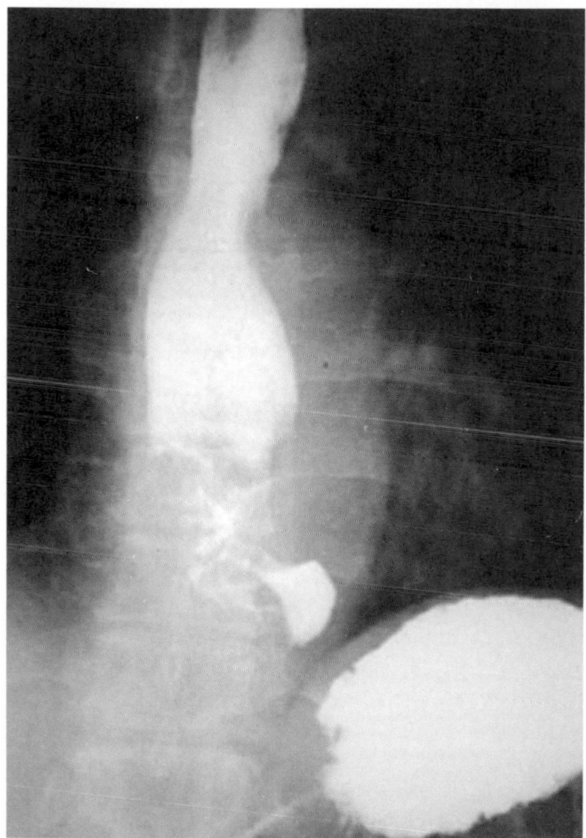

1. What is the finding?
2. What are some possible etiologies for the finding?
3. What finding is present on the upper GI examination?
4. In the absence of instrumentation, what is the most likely cause of the finding?

CASE 83

Hydropneumopericardium

1. Hydropneumopericardium.
2. Previous pericardiocentesis or pericardial window, esophagopericardial fistula.
3. A fungating mass consistent with esophageal carcinoma.
4. Esophagopericardial fistula.

References

Kaufman J, Thongsuwan N, Stern E, Karmy-Jones R. Esophageal-pericardial fistula with purulent pericarditis secondary to esophageal carcinoma presenting with tamponade. *Ann Thorac Surg* 75:288–289, 2003.

Meltzer P, Elkayam U, Parsons K, Gazzaniga A. Esophageal-pericardial fistula presenting as pericarditis. *Am Heart J* 105:148–150, 1983.

Comment

The chest radiographs reveal hydropneumopericardium. Given the lack of pericardial instrumentation and the presence of esophageal carcinoma, an esophagopericardial fistula is suspected. The diagnosis is confirmed by endoscopy.

Hydropneumopericardium usually occurs after pericardiocentesis or placement of a pericardial drain. Other causes, such as a fistula, are rare. Tumors that invade the pericardium include breast carcinoma, lung carcinoma, lymphoma, and esophageal carcinoma.

Notes

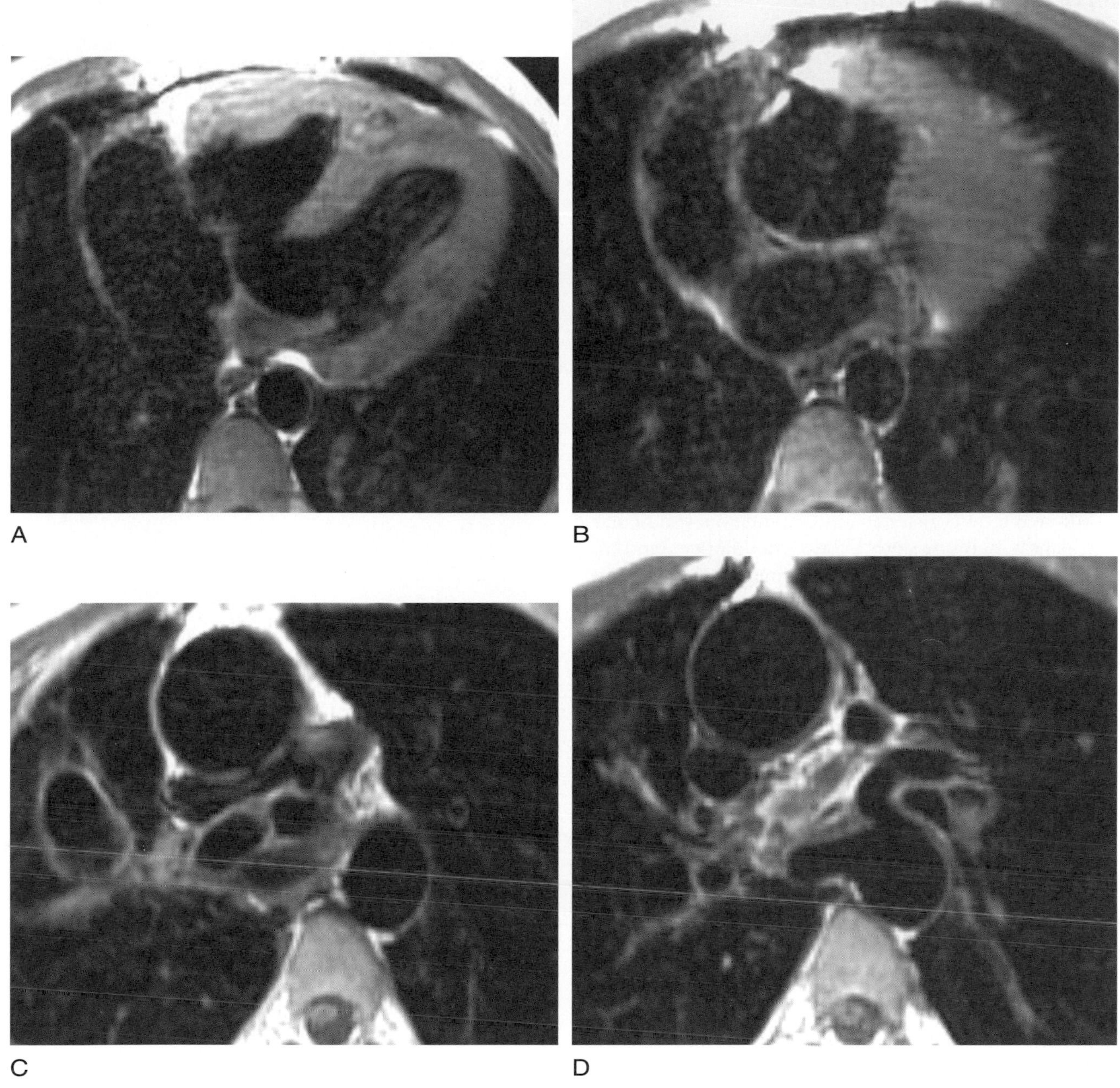

Axial spin-echo MR images.

1. Which intracardiac shunt is present?
2. Which chamber is hypertrophied?
3. How many great arteries arise from the heart (see Fig. B)?
4. What is the diagnosis?

CASE 84

Pulmonary Atresia with Ventricular Septal Defect

1. Ventricular septal defect.
2. Right ventricle.
3. One (aorta).
4. Pulmonary atresia with ventricular septal defect.

Reference

Reddy GP, Higgins CB. Magnetic resonance imaging of congenital heart disease: evaluation of morphology and function. *Semin Roentgenol* 38:342–351, 2003.

Cross-Reference

Cardiac Imaging: THE REQUISITES, 2nd edition, pp 351–353.

Comment

The MR image demonstrates a membraneous ventricular septal defect, hypertrophy of the right ventricle, and an overriding aorta (displaced to the right, over the septal defect). The aorta is the only great vessel that arises from the heart, thus indicating pulmonary atresia. These findings are consistent with pulmonary atresia with a ventricular septal defect. The central pulmonary arteries are hypoplastic (see Fig. C), and there are systemic-to-pulmonary arterial collaterals that arise from the descending aorta and supply the lungs (see Fig. D).

Pulmonary atresia with ventricular septal defect is a severe variant of tetralogy of Fallot. In the past, it was sometimes called "pseudotruncus," but it is important to remember that this anomaly is *not* a form of truncus arteriosus. The central pulmonary arteries are frequently hypoplastic, and the peripheral pulmonary arteries are often stenotic.

MRI is optimal for the assessment of the pulmonary arteries because it evaluates supracardiac structures more readily than does echocardiography and it does not rely on contrast enhancement to show the vessels, as does cineangiography. This is especially useful because the pulmonary arteries usually do not opacify well in the presence of pulmonary atresia.

Notes

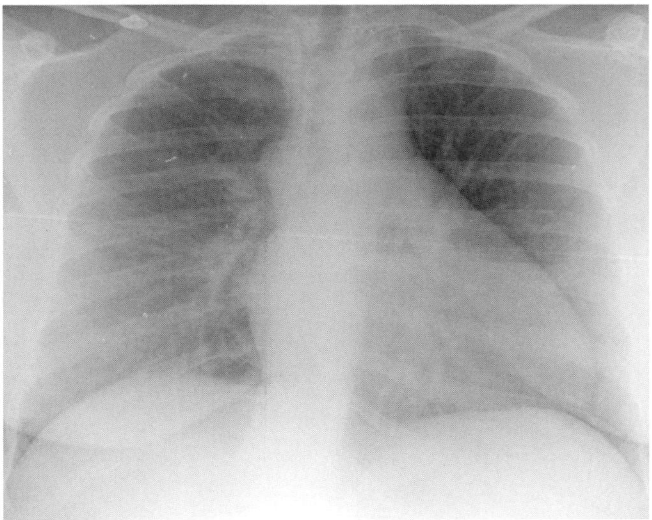

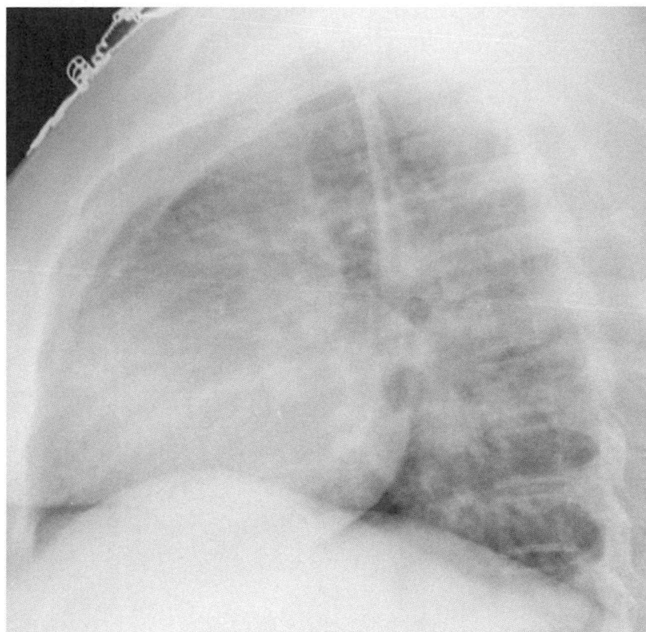

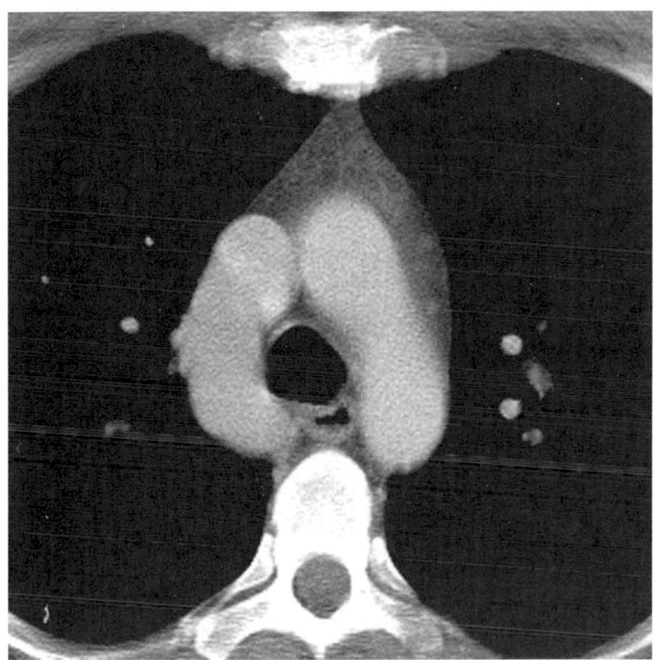

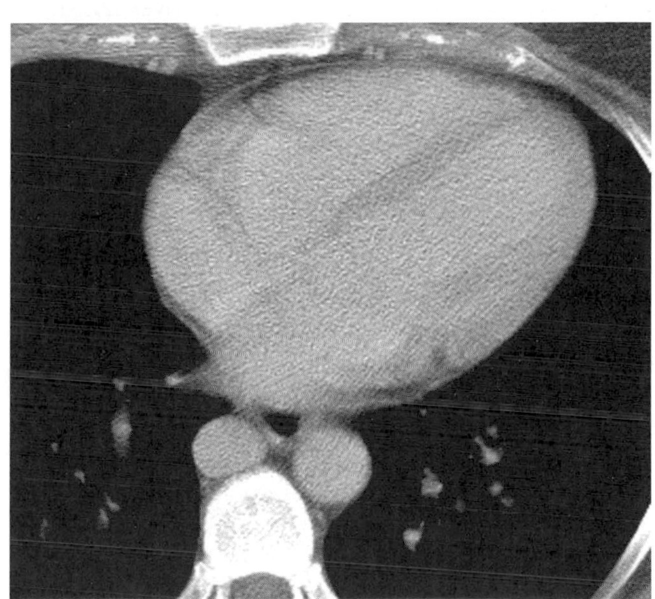

1. Which vessel is enlarged?
2. Which vessel is absent in the chest?
3. What is the diagnosis?
4. Which heterotaxic syndrome is associated with this lesion?

ANSWERS

CASE 85

Interruption of Inferior Vena Cava with Azygous Continuation

1. Azygous vein.
2. Inferior vena cava.
3. Interruption of the inferior vena cava with azygous continuation.
4. Bilateral left-sidedness/polysplenia syndrome.

Reference

Jelinek JS, Stuart PL, Done SL, Ghaed N, Rudd SA. MRI of polysplenia syndrome. *Magn Reson Imaging* 7:681–686, 1989.

Cross-Reference

Cardiac Imaging: THE REQUISITES, 2nd edition, p 297.

Comment

The plain films demonstrate no inferior vena cava shadow just above the diaphragm. The posteroanterior chest film and the CT images show marked enlargement of the azygous vein. This is consistent with interruption of the inferior vena cava with azygous continuation.

In this anomaly, the hepatic portion of the inferior vena cava is interrupted. Typically the blood passes through collateral channels to enter the azygous or hemizygous vein. The anomaly may be isolated, as in this case, or it may be associated with polysplenia syndrome.

Notes

CASE 86

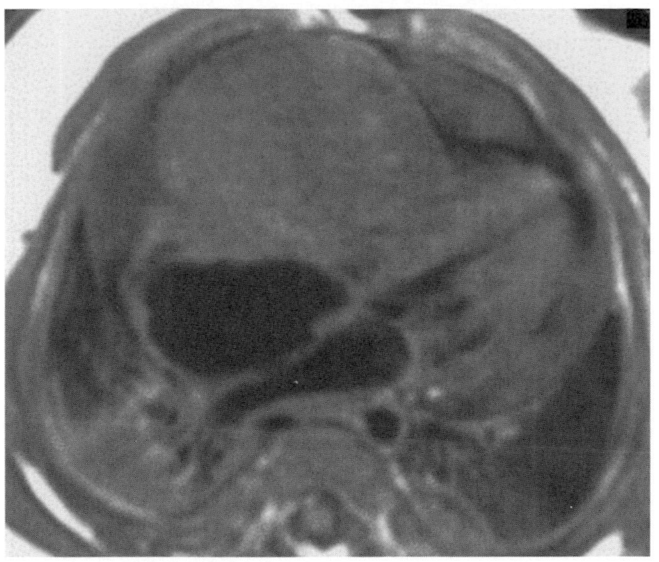

Axial spin-echo MR image.

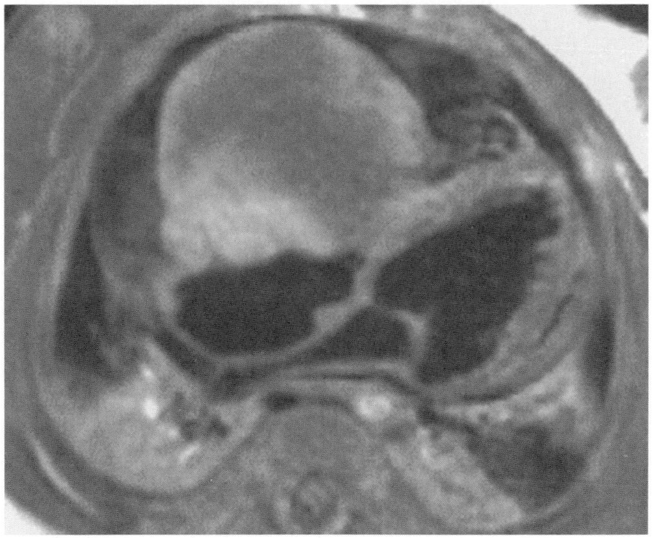

Axial spin-echo postgadolinium MR image with fat saturation.

1. Where is the mass centered?
2. Which chambers are compressed?
3. Is the mass benign or malignant?
4. What is the most likely diagnosis?

CASE 87

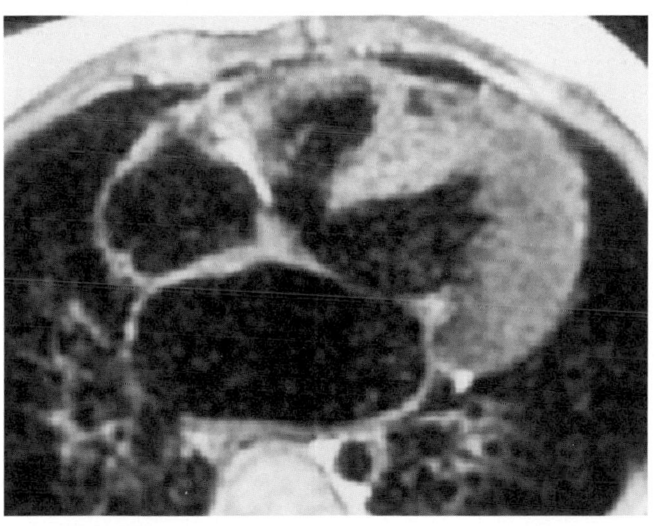

Axial spin-echo MR image.

Flow Rate (mL/sec)
500
450
400
350
300
250
200
150
100
50
0
1 2 3 4 5 6 7 8 9 10 11 12 13 14 15 16
Cardiac Phase

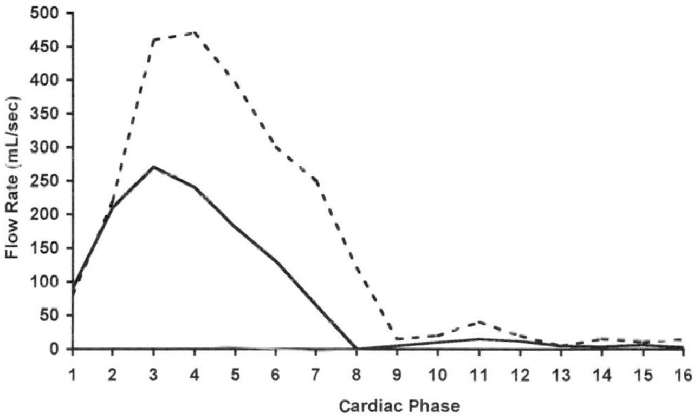

1. Which lesion does the patient have?
2. Which MRI sequence is most commonly used to measure blood flow?
3. What does the graph represent?
4. Why is pulmonary flow greater than systemic flow?

CASE 86

Cardiac Fibroma

1. Right ventricular free wall.
2. Right ventricle and right atrium.
3. Benign.
4. Fibroma.

Reference

Fujita N, Caputo GR, Higgins CB. Diagnosis and characterization of intracardiac masses by magnetic resonance imaging. *Am J Card Imaging* 8:69–80, 1994.

Cross-Reference

Cardiac Imaging: THE REQUISITES, 2nd edition, p 263.

Comment

Cardiac fibroma is a rare, benign tumor; approximately 90% occur in children. Fibromas are usually well-marginated masses that are mainly composed of spindle cells and intervening collagen. Microscopic calcification is present in approximately half these tumors.

MRI is useful for demonstration of tumor size and location and cardiac function. Contrast-enhanced MRI can delineate tumor margins and extension and involvement of adjacent structures. However, the presence of enhancement is not reliable for determination of malignancy. Features that suggest a primary malignant cardiac tumor include invasiveness, extension outside the heart, involvement of more than one chamber, central necrosis or cavitation, and large pericardial effusion. Absence of these findings indicates benignity.

The appearance of fibroma is variable on spin-echo T1-weighted images and cine-MRI. Because fibroma is often isointense to myocardium, the administration of contrast agent may be necessary to define the extent of tumor. Fibromas have been reported to show irregular peripheral enhancement or heterogeneous enhancement with dark areas corresponding to calcification. Because gadolinium chelate contrast agent equilibrates rapidly into the extracellular space, the peripheral enhancement pattern indicates poor vascularization of the central fibrous tissue. The periphery of the mass is better vascularized and has a larger extracellular space.

Since this enhancement pattern is comparable to that of a fast-growing tumor with central necrosis, it is not diagnostic of a fibroma. Definitive diagnosis requires endomyocardial or open biopsy, but MRI can be used to suggest the diagnosis of fibroma. Surgical resection is performed if the mass causes hemodynamic compromise.

Notes

CASE 87

Ventricular Septal Defect, with Flow Measurements

1. Ventricular septal defect.
2. Velocity-encoded cine phase-contrast MRI.
3. Pulmonary and systemic flow rates during the cardiac cycle.
4. Because there is a left-to-right shunt.

Reference

Varaprasathan GA, Araoz PA, Higgins CB, Reddy GP. Quantification of flow dynamics in congenital heart disease: applications of velocity-encoded cine MR imaging. *Radiographics* 22:895–905, 2002.

Cross-Reference

Cardiac Imaging: THE REQUISITES, 2nd edition, p 122.

Comment

The MR image shows a ventricular septal defect.

Velocity-encoded cine-MRI can be used to quantify intracardiac shunts. Velocity-encoded cine-MRI is used to measure blood flow in the pulmonary artery (pulmonary flow) and in the ascending aorta (systemic flow). Flow curves are obtained (see graph), and the curves are integrated to obtain flow per unit time. In the normal individual, the pulmonary-to-systemic flow ratio is 1 to 1. However, in a patient with a left-to-right shunt, the ratio is greater than 1. Operative repair may be beneficial when the flow ratio exceeds the range of 1.7 to 1.

Echocardiography is the mainstay of the imaging evaluation of cardiac shunts. However, MRI has an important role in shunt quantification and in the assessment of lesions such as supracristal ventricular septal defect and partial anomalous pulmonary venous return, for which echocardiographic evaluation may be limited.

Notes

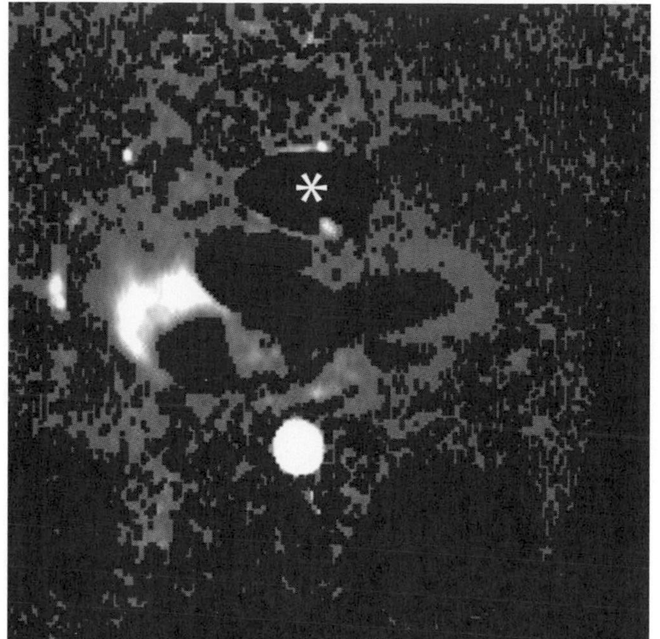

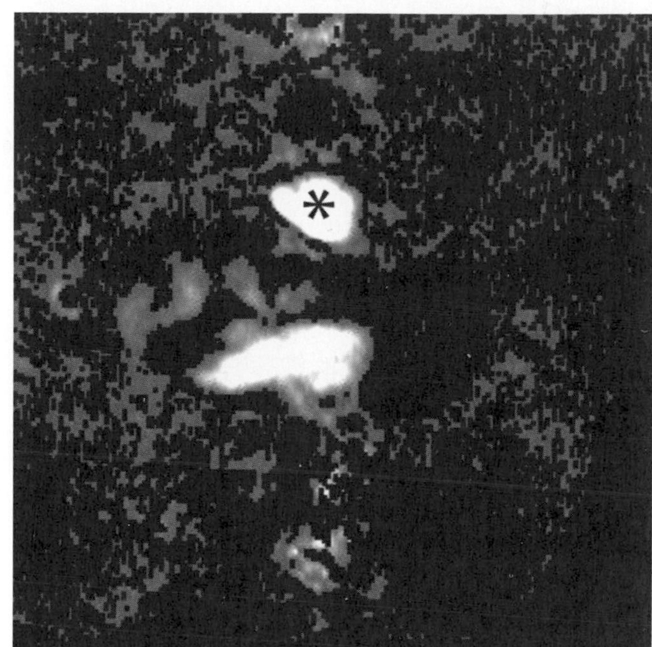

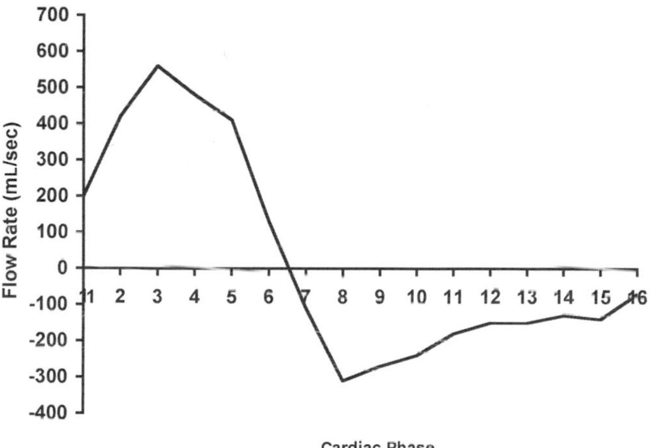

1. What MRI sequence is depicted in the images?
2. What structure is labeled with an asterisk (*)?
3. The patient has a history of tetralogy of Fallot, which was repaired in infancy. What is the diagnosis?
4. What does the graph represent?

CASE 88

Pulmonary Regurgitation after Repair of Tetralogy of Fallot

1. Velocity-encoded cine-MRI: phase images.
2. Pulmonary artery.
3. Pulmonary regurgitation.
4. The systolic portion of the graph depicts positive (antegrade) flow, and the diastolic portion shows negative (retrograde) flow.

Reference

Varaprasathan GA, Araoz PA, Higgins CB, Reddy GP. Quantification of flow dynamics in congenital heart disease: applications of velocity-encoded cine MR imaging. *Radiographics* 22:895–905, 2002.

Cross-Reference

Cardiac Imaging: THE REQUISITES, 2nd edition, p 193.

Comment

The velocity-encoded cine-MRI phase images show a forward flow (dark signal) in the pulmonary artery during systole and retrograde flow (bright signal) during diastole, indicating regurgitation. The flow curve represents a quantitative depiction of the same information.

Patients with tetralogy of Fallot typically undergo repair during infancy or early childhood. Frequently, the pulmonary infundibular stenosis is relieved by right ventriculoplasty. This procedure can cause long-term pulmonary valve insufficiency. Patients with pulmonary regurgitation may require replacement of the valve.

MRI is an ideal method to evaluate pulmonary regurgitation because this modality is noninvasive, does not require ionizing radiation, evaluates the right ventricle more readily than does echocardiography, and can accurately quantify pulmonary regurgitation and right ventricular volume.

Notes

CASE 89

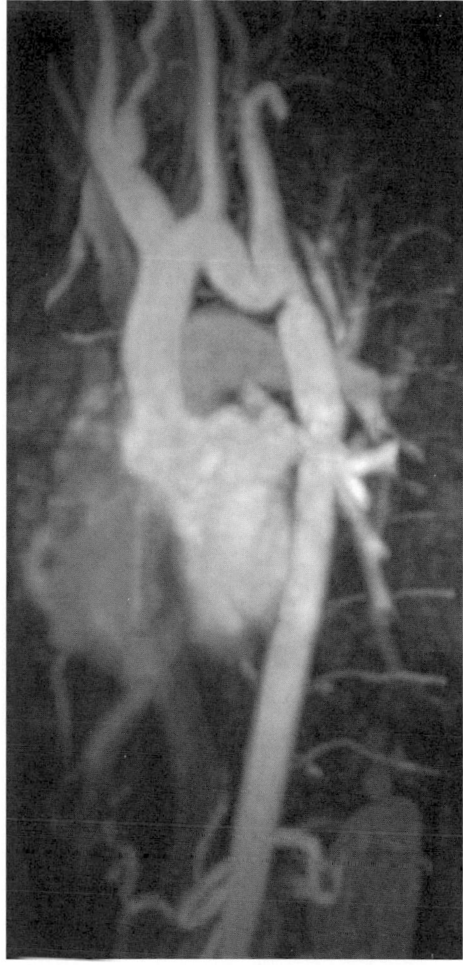

Flow Rate (mL/sec)

70 60 50 40 30 20 10 0

1 2 3 4 5 6 7 8 9 10 11 12 13 14 15 16

Cardiac Phase

Maximum-intensity projection of gadolinium-enhanced MR angiogram.

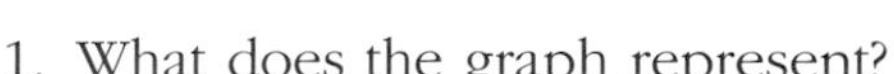

1. What does the graph represent?
2. What is the diagnosis?
3. Is the lesion hemodynamically significant?
4. In a young adult, how should this lesion be managed?

CASE 89

Coarctation of the Aorta, with Collateral Flow Measurements

1. The flow versus time curves indicate that flow in the distal aorta is greater than that in the proximal aorta. The difference in flow between the two locations is equal to the volume of collateral flow.
2. Coarctation of the aorta.
3. Yes.
4. Surgery or balloon angioplasty and stenting.

Reference

Varaprasathan GA, Araoz PA, Higgins CB, Reddy GP. Quantification of flow dynamics in congenital heart disease: applications of velocity-encoded cine MR imaging. *Radiographics* 22:895–905, 2002.

Cross-Reference

Cardiac Imaging: THE REQUISITES, 2nd edition, pp 117–119.

Comment

The MR angiogram demonstrates a discrete, juxtaductal coarctation of the aorta. No visible collateral vessels are noted. The flow versus time curves show that there is collateral circulation. The presence of collateral flow shows that the lesion is hemodynamically significant, even in the absence of visible collateral vessels.

In normal individuals, flow in the distal thoracic aorta is slightly lower than in the proximal descending aorta because the intercostal arteries and other aortic branches take blood away from the aorta. However, in a patient with a functionally significant coarctation, collateral vessels bring blood into the descending thoracic aorta and the distal flow is greater than the proximal flow.

Velocity-encoded cine-MRI is the only noninvasive method that can accurately quantify collateral circulation in coarctation of the aorta.

Notes

CASE 90

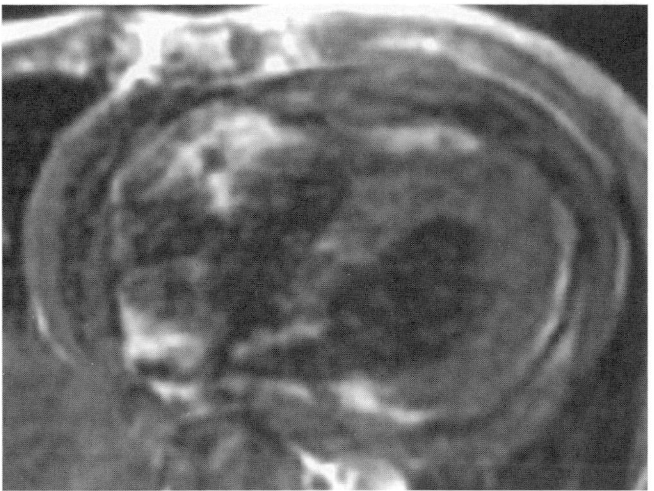

Axial spin-echo MR image.

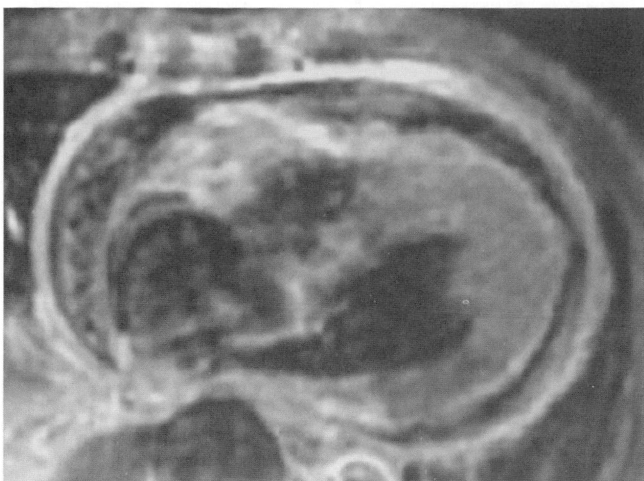

Axial spin-echo postgadolinium MR image with fat saturation.

1. Is the pericardial effusion simple or complex?
2. Which pericardial abnormalities are present?
3. In the setting of dyspnea, lower extremity edema, pleural effusions, and ascites, what is the diagnosis?
4. What is the most common etiology worldwide?

CASE 91

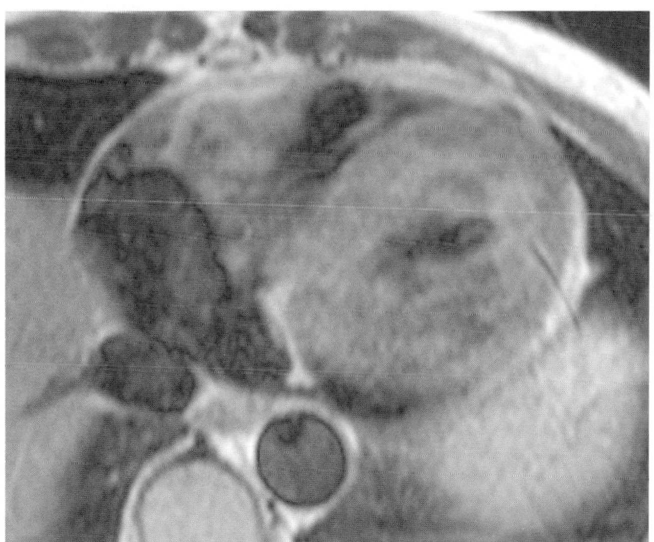

Axial spin-echo MR image.

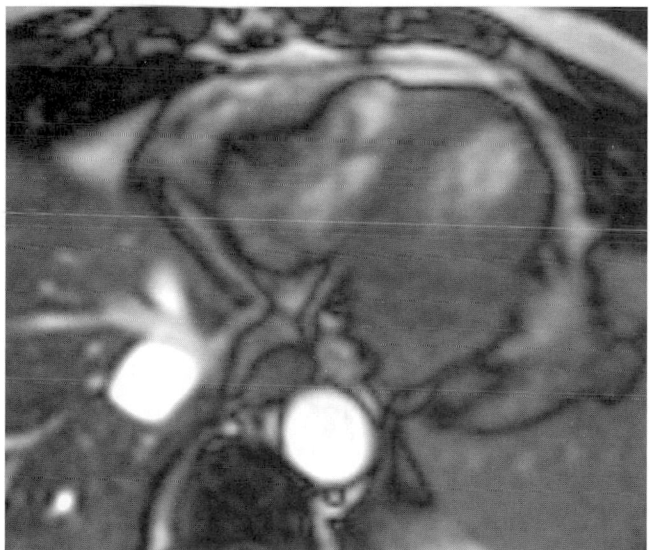

Axial gradient-echo cine-MR image.

1. What is the abnormality of the right ventricle?
2. The patient has an arrhythmia attributable to the right ventricle. What is the most likely diagnosis?
3. What other MRI findings can be seen in this disease?
4. Is there a genetic predisposition to this disease?

CASE 90

Effusive Constrictive Pericarditis

1. Complex.
2. Pericardial thickening (≥4 mm) and enhancement.
3. Effusive constrictive pericarditis.
4. Tuberculosis.

Reference

Wang ZJ, Reddy GP, Gotway MB, Yeh BM, Hetts SW, Higgins CB. CT and MR imaging of pericardial disease. *Radiographics* 23(Special Issue):S167–S180, 2003.

Cross-Reference

Cardiac Imaging: THE REQUISITES, 2nd edition, pp 253–256.

Comment

This patient has a complex pericardial effusion, as well as pericardial thickening and enhancement. In the setting of constrictive/restrictive physiology, the diagnosis is effusive constrictive pericarditis.

Pericardiocentesis can relieve the acute illness, but chronic constrictive pericarditis can develop. The patient underwent pericardiocentesis, and the fluid revealed acid-fast bacilli, which were identified on culture as *Mycobacterium tuberculosis.*

Notes

CASE 91

Arrhythmogenic Right Ventricular Dysplasia with a Right Ventricular Aneurysm

1. Focal wall thinning and bulging, consistent with an aneurysm. This demonstrated paradoxical motion on the Cine loop (not shown).
2. Arrhythmogenic right ventricular dysplasia.
3. Fatty infiltration of the right ventricular free wall.
4. Probably.

Reference

Bremerich J, Pater S, Buser PT. Magnetic resonance imaging of acquired heart disease: evaluation of structure. *Semin Roentgenol* 38:314–319, 2003.

Cross-Reference

Cardiac Imaging: THE REQUISITES, 2nd edition, pp 277–280.

Comment

Arrhythmogenic right ventricular dysplasia typically presents as ventricular tachycardia or tachyarrhythmia originating in the right ventricle. There is replacement of the right ventricular myocardium by fat or fibrous tissue.

The diagnosis of right ventricular dysplasia is established by clinical, electrophysiologic, echocardiographic, and MRI findings. Although MRI is a major diagnostic criterion, an abnormal MRI is neither necessary nor sufficient for the diagnosis. Approximately 50% of patients have a family history of the disease, although the genetic causes have not been definitively ascertained.

Spin-echo MR images can demonstrate fat in the right ventricular myocardium. Focal wall thinning and aneurysm are other findings that can be seen in this disease.

Notes

CASE 92

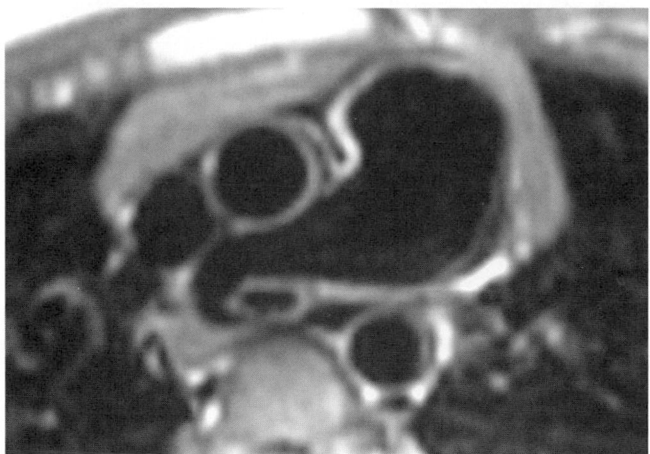

Axial spin-echo MR image.

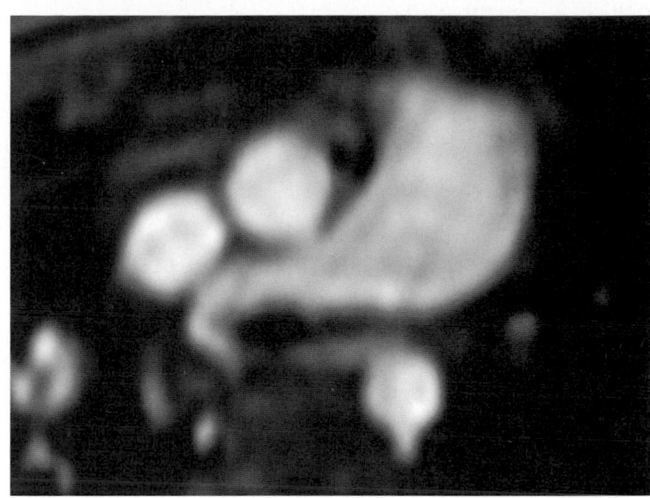

Axial gradient-echo cine-MR image.

1. Where does the left pulmonary artery originate?
2. What is the course of the left pulmonary artery?
3. What is the diagnosis?
4. What is the clinical significance of this lesion?

CASE 92

Pulmonary Sling

1. From the distal right pulmonary artery.
2. It passes posterior to the trachea and anterior to the esophagus. (The esophagus is not displayed on these images.)
3. Pulmonary sling.
4. This is a vascular ring that compresses the trachea and right mainstem bronchus to a variable degree. Because the left pulmonary artery is hypoplastic, there is reduced blood flow to the left lung.

Reference

Eichhorn J, Fink C, Bock M, Delorme S, Brockmeier K, Ulmer HE. Images in cardiovascular medicine: time-resolved three-dimensional magnetic resonance angiography for assessing a pulmonary artery sling in a pediatric patient. *Circulation* 106:E61–E62, 2002.

Cross-Reference

Cardiac Imaging: THE REQUISITES, 2nd edition, pp 408–410.

Comment

Pulmonary sling is a rare anomaly in which a hypoplastic left pulmonary artery arises from the distal right pulmonary artery and passes between the trachea and esophagus. The term sling refers to the loop around the airway formed by the left pulmonary artery. Patients have symptoms of airway compression: dyspnea and wheezing.

Dynamic expiratory CT can be used to evaluate the severity of airway compression, and velocity-encoded cine-MRI can be employed to assess differential flow in the left and right pulmonary arteries. In the patient discussed here, the right pulmonary artery received approximately 79% of pulmonary blood flow, and the left only 21%.

Notes

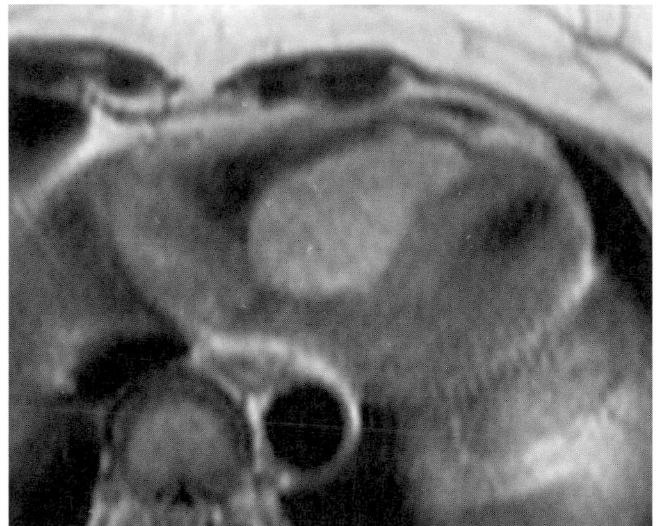
Axial spin-echo MR image.

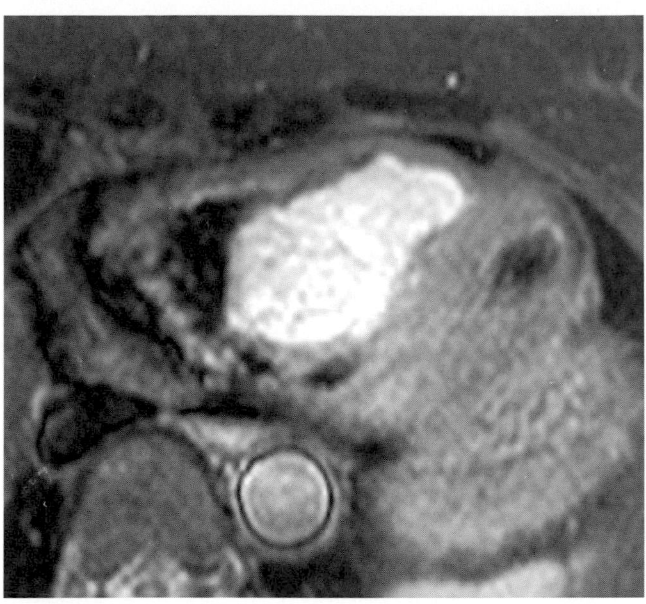
Axial spin-echo T2-weighted MR image with fat saturation.

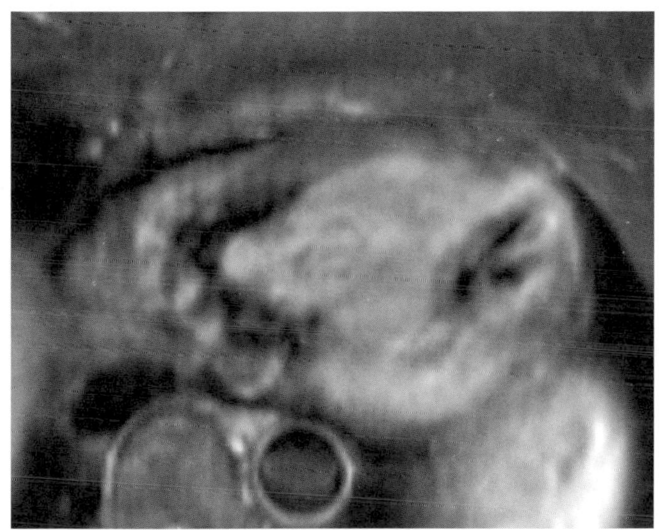
Axial spin-echo postgadolinium T1-weighted MR image with fat saturation.

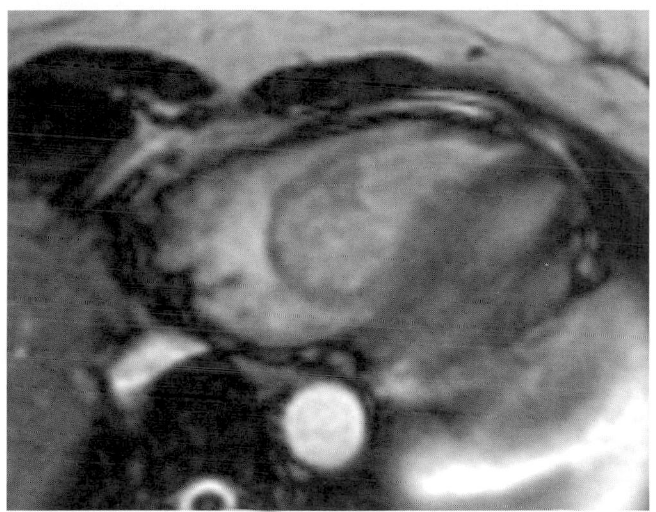
Axial gradient-echo cine-MR image.

1. Where is the mass centered?
2. What MRI features are suggestive of a malignant cardiac mass?
3. Is this mass malignant or benign?
4. What are the two most common benign tumors in the heart?

ANSWERS

CASE 93

Cardiac Hemangioma

1. Right ventricular chamber.
2. Extension outside of the heart, invasiveness, involvement of more than one chamber, central necrosis or cavitation, large pericardial effusion.
3. Benign.
4. Myxoma and lipoma.

Reference

Moniotte S, Geva T, Perez-Atayde A, Fulton DR, Pigula FA, Powell AJ. Images in cardiovascular medicine: cardiac hemangioma. *Circulation* 112:E103–E104, 2005.

Cross-Reference

Cardiac Imaging: THE REQUISITES, 2nd edition, p 266.

Comment

Hemangiomas are benign proliferations of endothelial cells and vessels. These masses can be classified as a cavernous, a capillary, or an arteriovenous subtype, depending on the dominant vascular channel. Hemangiomas can contain calcification, fat, and fibrous tissue. Cardiac hemangiomas are rare and can be intramural or within a chamber.

Clinical symptoms and signs include dyspnea on exertion, arrhythmia, angina, and right heart failure. Right ventricular outflow obstruction is the usual cause of dyspnea in patients with hemangioma.

CT can be used to delineate the location, size, and extent of the mass. On CT, a hemangioma is typically heterogeneous and often demonstrates areas of calcification. Iodinated contrast agent is useful to demonstrate marked enhancement of this vascular mass.

MRI can provide optimal evaluation of a cardiac mass. Hemangiomas demonstrate low-to-intermediate signal intensity on T1-weighted images and high signal intensity on T2-weighted images, but occasionally the mass shows high signal intensity on T1-weighted and images also.

When a mass demonstrates high signal intensity on T1-weighted images, it is important to consider the diagnoses of lipoma and melanoma in addition to hemangioma. Hemangiomas do not lose signal with fat suppression techniques, allowing differentiation from lipomas. Melanoma metastases and other malignant tumors are infiltrative, unlike a hemangioma.

Notes

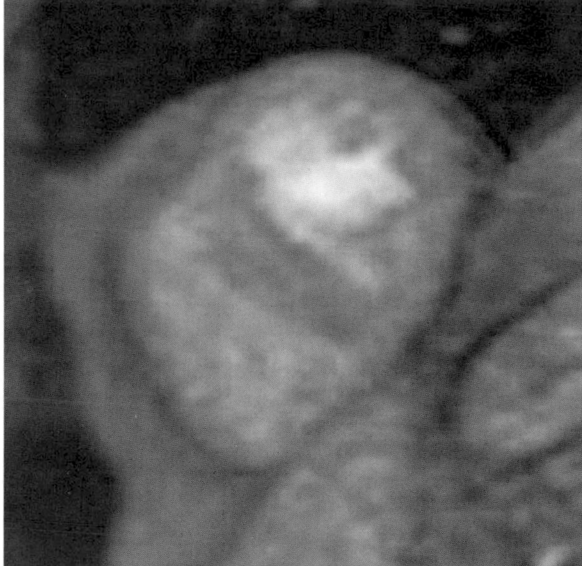

Short-axis first-pass perfusion MR image before treatment.

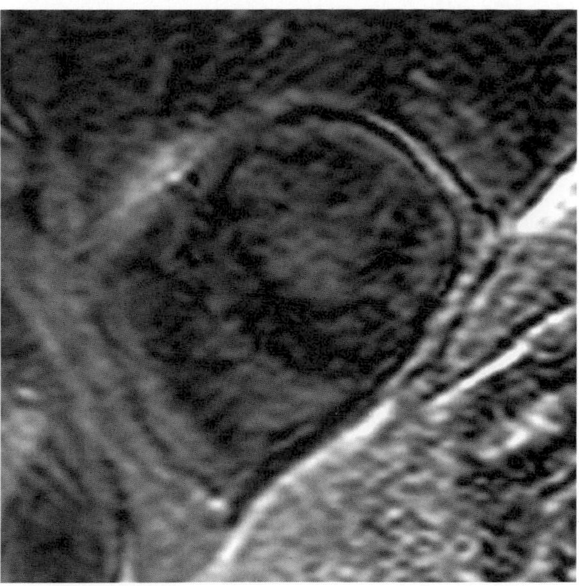

Short-axis delayed-enhancement MR image before treatment.

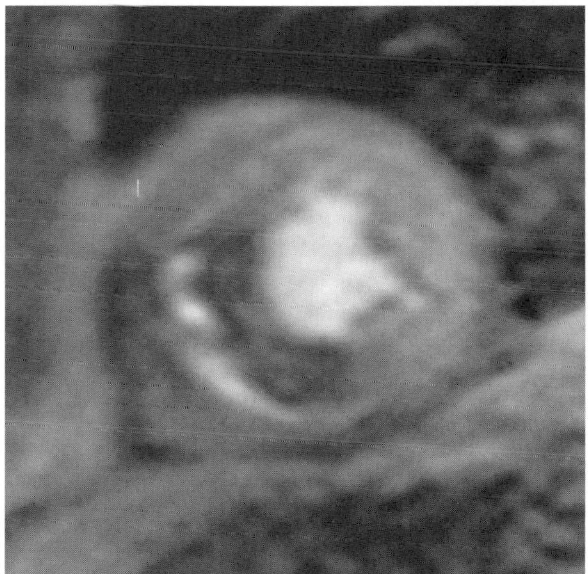

Short-axis first-pass perfusion MR image after treatment.

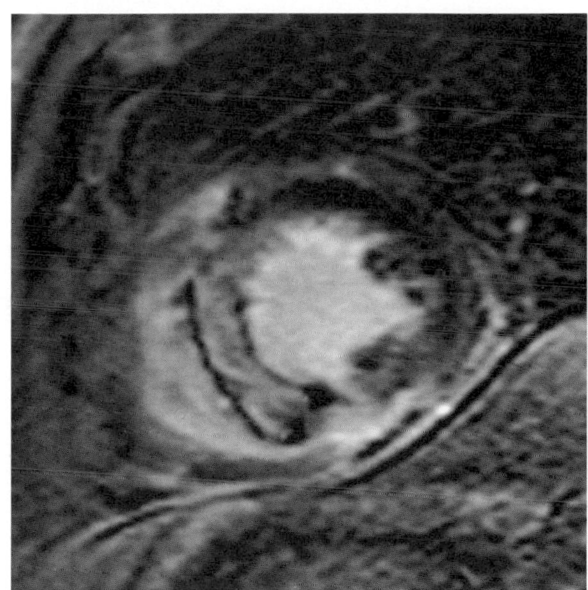

Short-axis delayed-enhancement MR image after treatment.

1. What does the posttreatment perfusion image show?
2. What abnormal signal intensity is seen on the posttreatment delayed-enhancement image?
3. What is the significance of this abnormal signal intensity?
4. The patient underwent minimally invasive therapy for hypertrophic cardiomyopathy. What was the therapy?

CASE 94

Hypertrophic Cardiomyopathy after Treatment

1. Hypoperfusion in the interventricular septum.
2. Hyperenhancement.
3. It indicates infarction.
4. Ethanol septal ablation.

Reference

Amano Y, Takayama M, Amano M, Kumazaki T. MRI of cardiac morphology and function after percutaneous transluminal septal myocardial ablation for hypertrophic obstructive cardiomyopathy. *AJR Am J Roentgenol* 182:523–527, 2004.

Cross-Reference

Cardiac Imaging: THE REQUISITES, 2nd edition, pp 100–102, 272–275.

Comment

Ethanol septal ablation has been developed in recent years for the treatment of hypertrophic cardiomyopathy with asymmetric septal hypertrophy, the most common form of hypertrophic cardiomyopathy. The MR image demonstrates septal infarction and hypoperfusion, which resulted from the ablation.

Notes

CASE 95

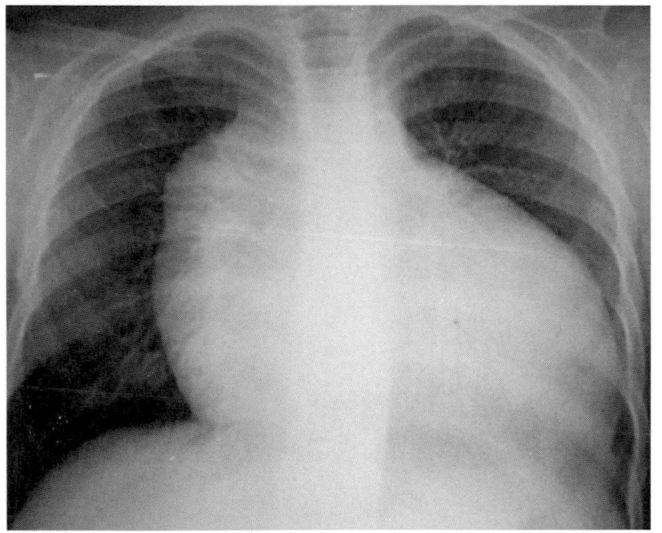

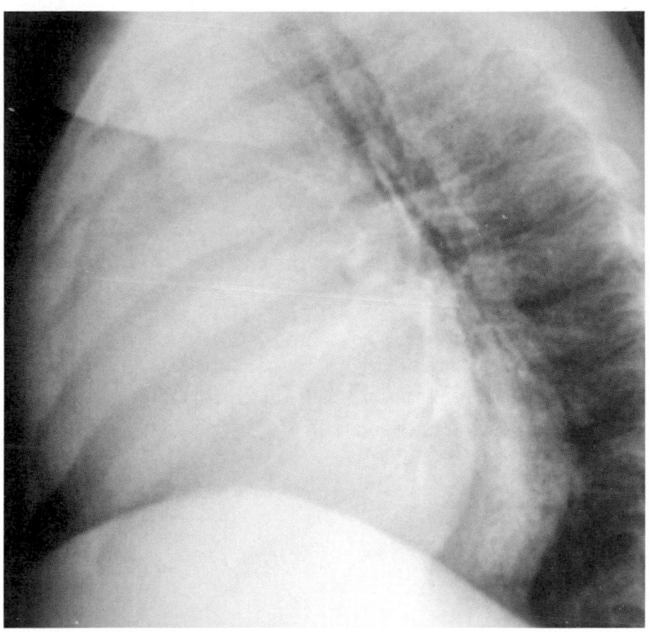

1. What are the abnormalities?
2. Would you expect this patient to be cyanotic?
3. The patient is 4 years old. What is the most likely diagnosis?
4. What is the differential diagnosis?

ANSWERS

CASE 95

Ebstein Anomaly

1. Decreased pulmonary vascularity and cardiomegaly.
2. Yes; the pulmonary blood flow is diminished.
3. Ebstein anomaly.
4. Critical pulmonary stenosis, pulmonary atresia with intact ventricular septum, and tricuspid atresia with a restrictive ventricular septal defect.

Reference

Higgins CB. Radiography of congenital heart disease. In Webb WR, Higgins CB, editors: *Thoracic imaging: pulmonary and cardiovascular radiology*. Philadelphia, 2005, Lippincott Williams & Wilkins, pp 679–706.

Cross-Reference

Cardiac Imaging: THE REQUISITES, 2nd edition, pp 198–200.

Comment

Ebstein anomaly is characterized by an abnormality of the tricuspid valve: the septal and posterior leaflets are displaced apically, causing tricuspid regurgitation. A portion of the right ventricle is functionally incorporated into the atrium, which is known as "atrialization of the right ventricle" although the atrialized portion of the ventricle contracts during ventricular systole.

Tricuspid regurgitation causes marked enlargement of the right ventricle and atrium. Tricuspid regurgitation with a coexisting atrial septal defect will result in a right-to-left shunt. Therefore, pulmonary vascularity is decreased and cyanosis can develop.

Notes

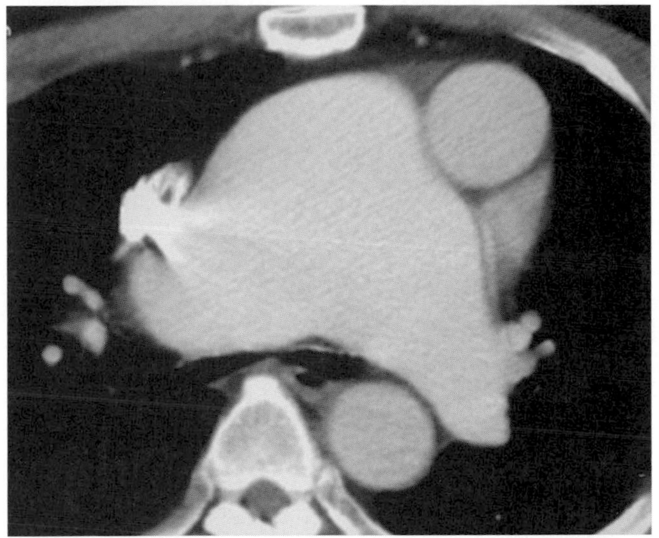

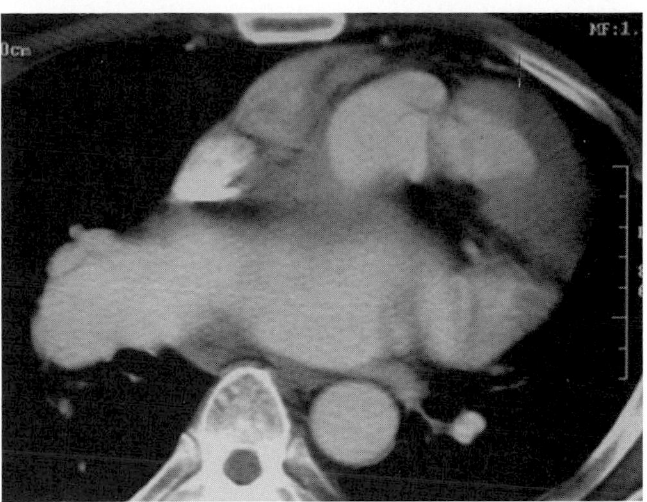

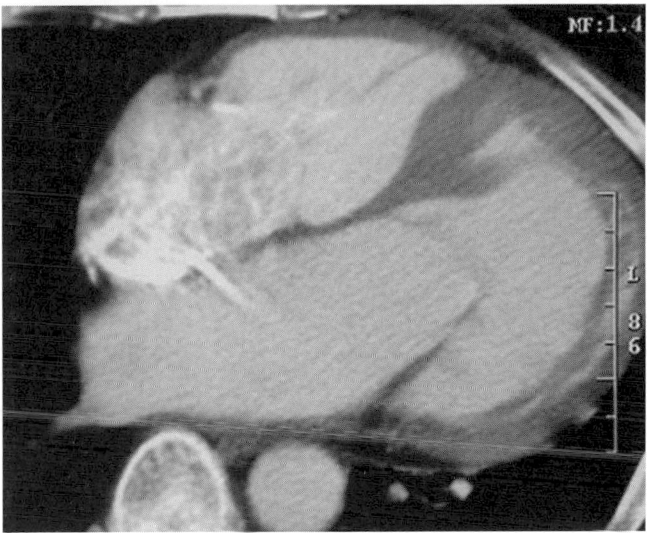

1. What is the relationship of the ascending aorta to the main pulmonary artery?
2. What are four characteristic features of the right ventricle?
3. Which ventricle gives rise to the aorta?
4. What is the most likely diagnosis?

CASE 96

Congenitally Corrected Transposition of the Great Arteries

1. The aorta is to the left of and slightly anterior to the main pulmonary artery.
2. The right ventricle has a muscular infundibulum, a moderator band, a heavily trabecular apex, and separation of the inflow and outflow valves.
3. Right ventricle.
4. Congenitally corrected transposition of the great arteries.

Reference

Hoeffel JC. Congenitally corrected transposition of the great arteries (L-TGA) with situs inversus totalis in adulthood: findings with magnetic resonance imaging. *Magn Reson Imaging* 19:762, 2001.

Cross-Reference

Cardiac Imaging: THE REQUISITES, 2nd edition, pp 298–301.

Comment

The CT scan shows the ascending aorta to the left and slightly anterior to the location of the pulmonary artery. The aorta arises from the ventricle that has a muscular infundibulum and a moderator band (the right ventricle, which in this patient is located on the left side of the heart). The right atrium receives the inferior vena cava (not shown) and connects to the left ventricle. The left atrium connects to the right ventricle. These findings are consistent with congenitally corrected transposition of the great arteries. Note that this patient also has marked pulmonary artery enlargement.

In congenitally corrected transposition of the great arteries, blood flows in the appropriate direction, and if no other abnormalities exist, patients may be asymptomatic. However, coexistent abnormalities may dominate the clinical picture in more than 90% of patients. Associated anomalies include the Ebstein malformation, ventricular septal defect, and supravalvular pulmonary stenosis. Patients with these lesions usually are symptomatic in infancy or early childhood.

Notes

CASE 97

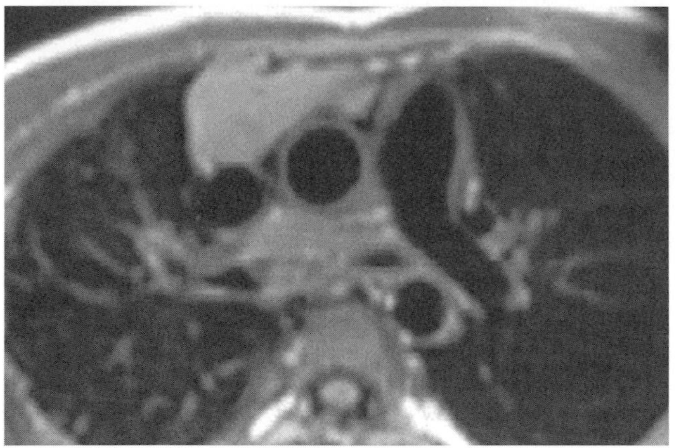

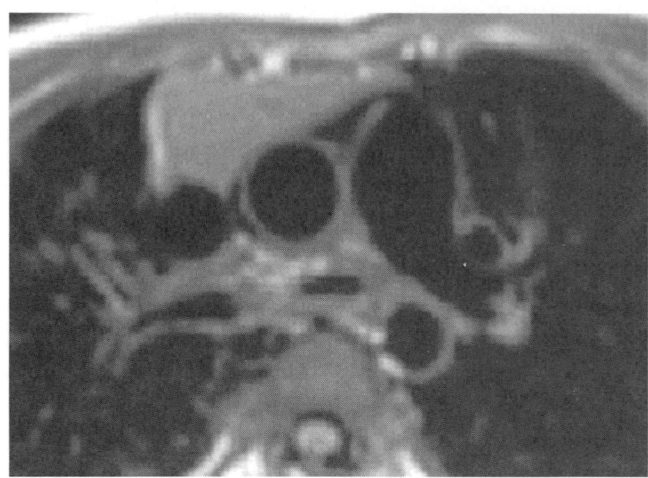

Axial spin-echo MR images.

1. Which structure is absent?
2. Is the anomaly ipsilateral or contralateral to the aortic arch?
3. How does the affected lung receive blood flow?
4. Is the affected lung usually hypoplastic?

CASE 98

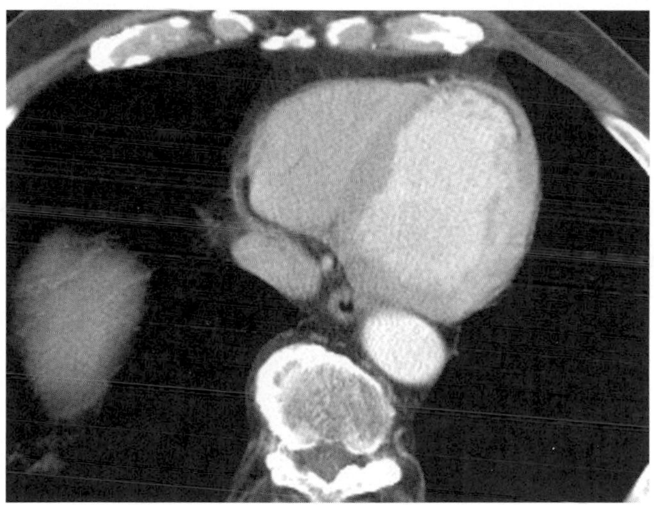

1. What abnormalities are noted in the left ventricular apex?
2. What is the etiology of the abnormalities?
3. What abnormality of wall motion would you expect?
4. What studies can be performed to assess myocardial viability?

CASE 97

"Absent" Right Pulmonary Artery

1. The proximal right pulmonary artery.
2. Contralateral.
3. Via systemic-to-pulmonary collateral arteries.
4. Yes.

References

Hernandez RJ. Magnetic resonance imaging of mediastinal vessels. Magn *Reson Imaging Clin N Am* 10:237–251, 2002.

Zylak CJ, Eyler WR, Spizarny DL, Stone CH. Developmental lung anomalies in the adult: radiologic-pathologic correlation. *Radiographics* 22(Special Issue):S25–S43, 2002.

Comment

Proximal interruption of, or "absent," pulmonary artery is a rare anomaly that occurs contralateral to the aortic arch. Although the proximal segment of the pulmonary artery is absent, there is a rudimentary artery in the hilum. The affected lung is usually hypoplastic, and it receives blood flow via systemic-to-pulmonary collateral channels. The diagnosis depends on the lack of visualization of the artery on echocardiography, CT, or MRI.

Notes

CASE 98

Myocardial Perfusion Defect

1. Wall thinning and subendocardial hypoperfusion.
2. Prior myocardial infarction.
3. Hypokinesis, akinesis, or dyskinesis.
4. Delayed-enhancement MRI or positron emission tomography (PET).

Reference

Pujadas S, Reddy GP, Lee JJ, Higgins CB. Magnetic resonance imaging in ischemic heart disease. *Semin Roentgenol* 38:320–329, 2003.

Cross-Reference

Cardiac Imaging: THE REQUISITES, 2nd edition, pp 98–100.

Comment

Myocardial wall thinning usually is a consequence of infarction. Subendocardial hypoperfusion could reflect ischemic or infarcted tissue. Relatively little work has been performed to investigate the utility of CT myocardial perfusion imaging. The affected area likely has diminished contractile function.

Delayed-enhancement MRI or PET can be performed to assess viability. If viable tissue is present in the area of functional abnormality, the patient could benefit from a revascularization procedure such as balloon angioplasty or coronary artery bypass graft surgery.

Notes

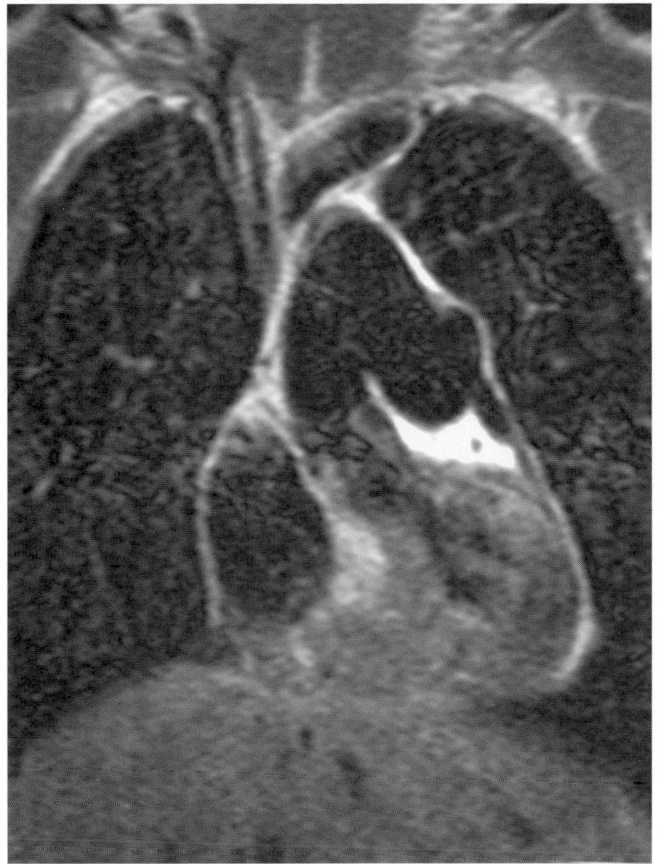

Coronal spin-echo MR image.

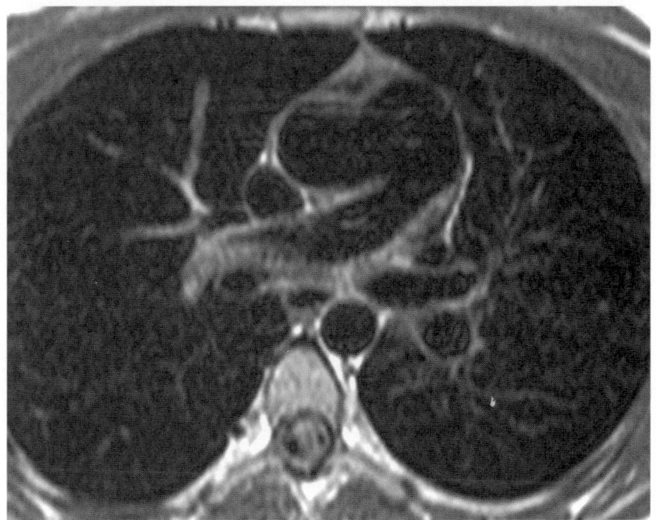

Axial spin-echo MR image.

1. Which two structures demonstrate an abnormal connection?
2. What is the name of the anomaly?
3. In an infant, in what direction would you expect blood to flow across the lesion?
4. Velocity-encoded cine-MRI showed that the pulmonary-to-systemic flow ratio in this patient was 0.9 to 1. What is the explanation?

ANSWERS

CASE 99

Eisenmenger Syndrome Secondary to Cardiovascular Shunt—Aorticopulmonary Window

1. The ascending aorta and main pulmonary artery.
2. Aorticopulmonary window.
3. From left to right.
4. The shunt reversed direction as a consequence of pulmonary hypertension.

Reference

Wang ZJ, Reddy GP, Gotway MB, Yeh BM, Higgins CB. Cardiovascular shunts: MR imaging evaluation. *Radiographics* 23(Special Issue):S181–S194, 2003.

Cross-Reference

Cardiac Imaging: THE REQUISITES, 2nd edition, pp 23–26.

Comment

Aorticopulmonary window is a rare anomaly in which there is a connection between the ascending aorta and the main pulmonary artery. This is a left-to-right shunt in infants and young children. Longstanding shunting can cause pulmonary hypertension and can lead to reversal of the shunt, a condition known as Eisenmenger syndrome.

Velocity-encoded cine-MRI can be used to assess the direction and severity of the shunt.

Notes

CASE 100

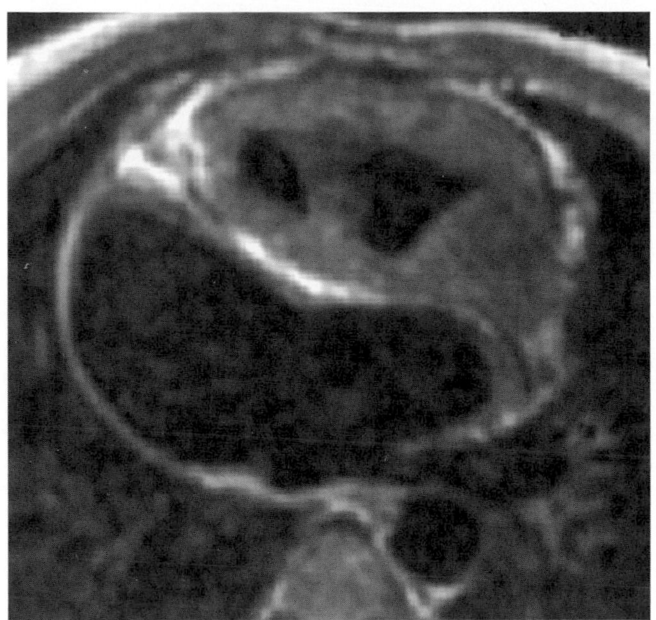

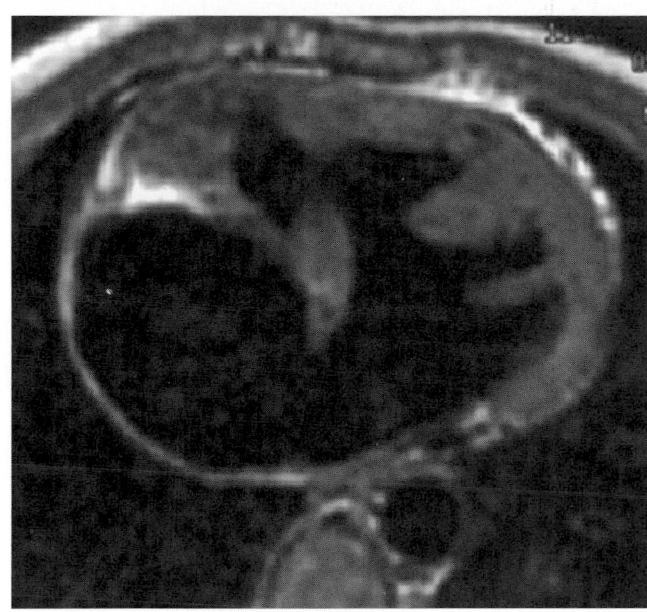

Axial spin-echo MR images.

1. In this patient, which great arteries arise from a muscular infundibulum?
2. What is the diagnosis?
3. What other anomalies are present?
4. Would you expect the patient to be cyanotic?

CASE 100

Double-Outlet Right Ventricle

1. The aorta and pulmonary artery.
2. Double-outlet right ventricle. A muscular infundibulum at the base of an artery indicates connection to the right ventricle.
3. Common atrium and large ventricular septal defect.
4. Yes.

Reference

Reddy GP, Higgins CB. Magnetic resonance imaging of congenital heart disease: evaluation of morphology and function. *Semin Roentgenol* 38:342–351, 2003.

Cross-Reference

Cardiac Imaging: THE REQUISITES, 2nd edition, pp 305–309.

Comment

Double-outlet right ventricle is a rare admixture lesion that causes shunt vascularity and cyanosis. The diagnosis is made by ascertaining that both great arteries arise from a muscular infundibulum, indicating a right ventricular origin. Atrial and ventricular septal defects usually coexist with this anomaly.

MRI readily demonstrates the pathologic anatomy and is therefore the ideal imaging modality for the diagnosis of double-outlet right ventricle.

Notes

CASE 101

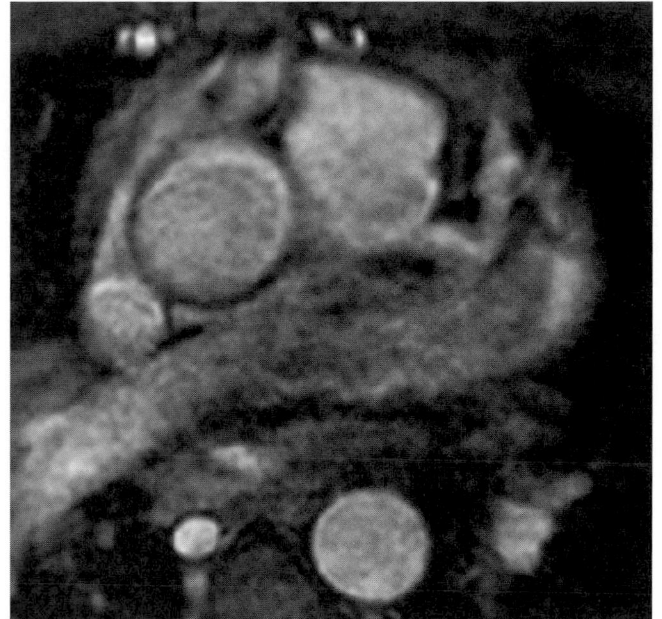

Axial gradient-echo cine-MR image.

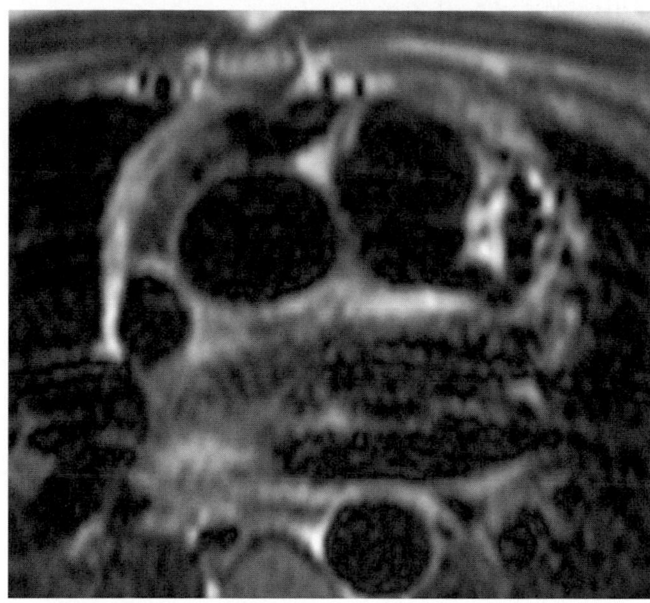

Axial spin-echo MR image.

1. What coronary anomaly is present?
2. Which symptoms do patients usually have?
3. What is the direction of blood flow in the left coronary artery?
4. What is the cause of ischemia in patients with this anomaly?

CASE 101

Anomalous Left Coronary Artery Arising from Pulmonary Artery

1. Anomalous left coronary artery arising from the pulmonary artery.
2. Failure to thrive and a high-pitched cry during feeding.
3. Toward the pulmonary artery. In other words, the flow is reversed.
4. Coronary steal phenomenon.

Reference

Bruder O, Sabin GV, Barkhausen J. Magnetic resonance imaging of anomalous origin of the left coronary artery from the pulmonary artery (Bland-White-Garland syndrome). *Heart* 91:656, 2005.

Cross-Reference

Cardiac Imaging: THE REQUISITES, 2nd edition, p 223.

Comment

Anomalous origin of the left coronary artery from the pulmonary artery is a rare lesion that usually presents during early infancy with failure to thrive and high-pitched crying during feeding. In response to ischemia, collateral vessels develop between the right and left coronary trees. Because the pulmonary circulation is a low-pressure system, blood is shunted from the coronary artery into the pulmonary artery, a phenomenon known as coronary steal. Early surgical correction is necessary because most untreated patients experience ischemia and myocardial infarction and develop ischemic cardiomyopathy within the first few years of life.

Echocardiography usually establishes the diagnosis, but sometimes angiography, MRI, or CT may be necessary to confirm the type of anomaly.

Notes

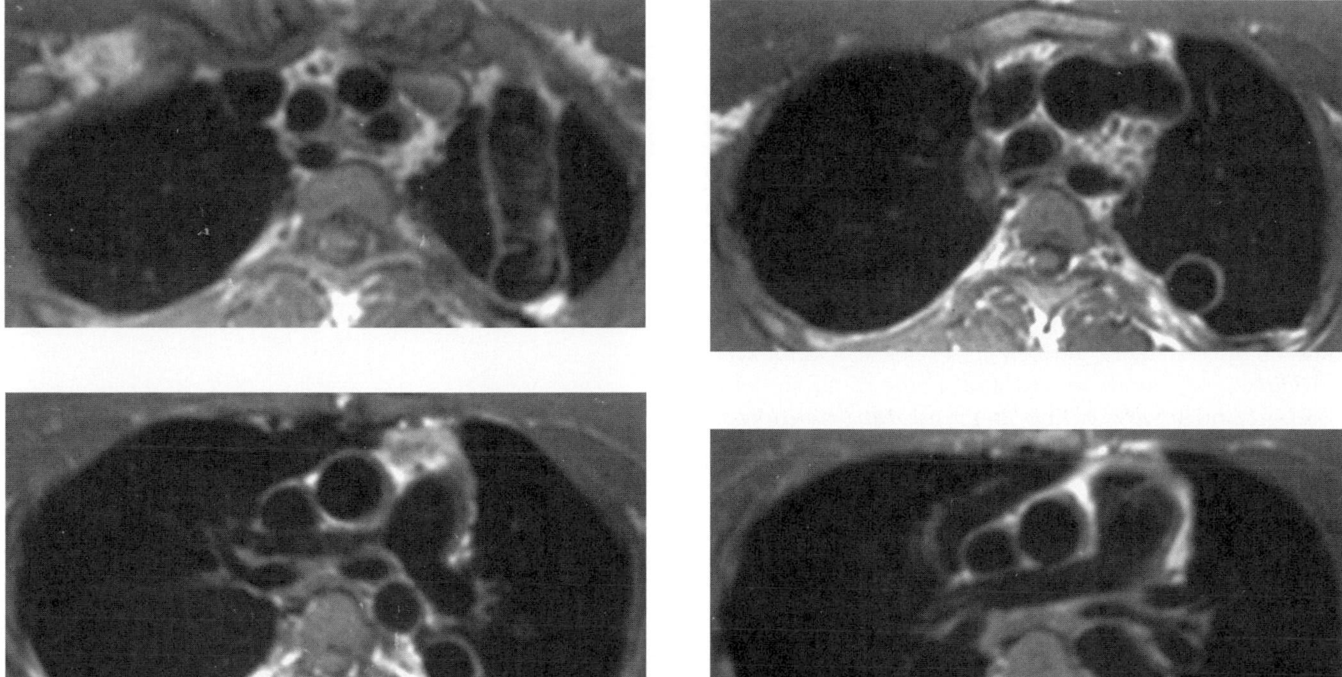

Axial spin-echo MR images.

1. Which surgery was performed?
2. What was the original lesion?
3. How do the lower extremities receive blood flow in the original lesion?
4. Is oxygen saturation normal in the lower extremity arteries?

CASE 102

Interrupted Aortic Arch with Bypass Surgery

1. Bypass graft between the ascending aorta and the descending aorta.
2. Interruption of the aortic arch.
3. Via a patent ductus arteriosus.
4. No; it is decreased.

Reference

Akdemir R, Ozhan H, Erbilen E, Yazici M, Gunduz H, Uyan C. Isolated interrupted aortic arch: a case report and review of the literature. *Int J Cardiovasc Imaging* 20:389–392, 2004.

Cross-Reference

Cardiac Imaging: THE REQUISITES, 2nd edition, pp 420–425.

Comment

Interrupted aortic arch occurs in three forms: the arch interruption can be located distal to the left subclavian artery origin (type A), proximal to the left subclavian artery (type B), or between the brachiocephalic and left common carotid arteries (type C). The descending aorta receives its blood flow from the pulmonary circulation via a patent ductus arteriosus. Therefore, arterial oxygen saturation is diminished in the abdominal and lower extremity arteries. Prostaglandin therapy should be administered to maintain patency of the ductus, which is vital. Bypass surgery usually is performed during infancy.

Notes

CASE 103

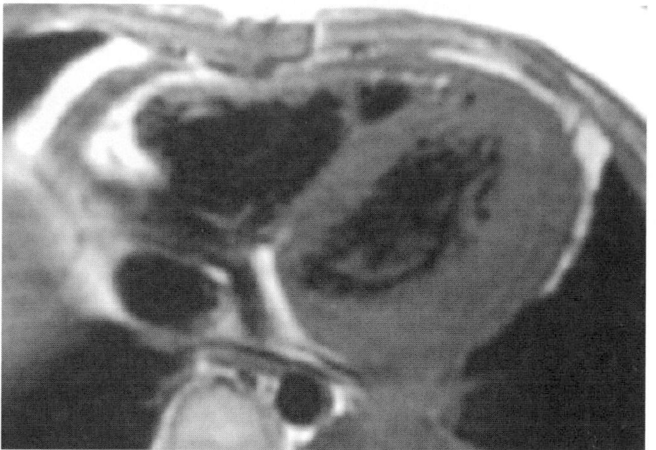

Axial spin-echo MR image.

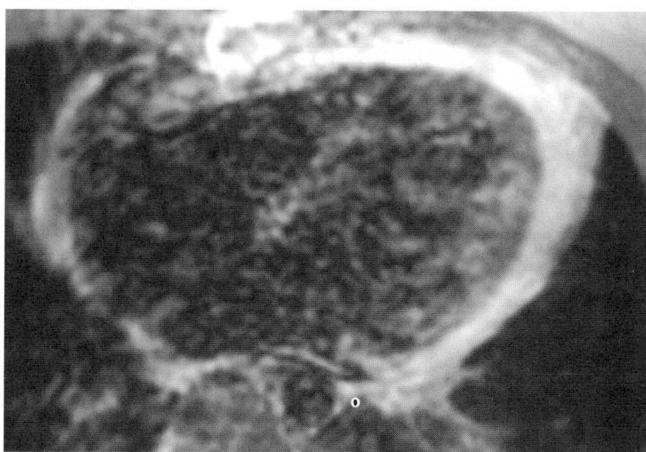

Axial spin-echo postgadolinium MR image with fat saturation.

1. What pericardial abnormalities are present?
2. What structure is enhancing intensely?
3. In the setting of constriction, what is the diagnosis?
4. What is the treatment?

CASE 104

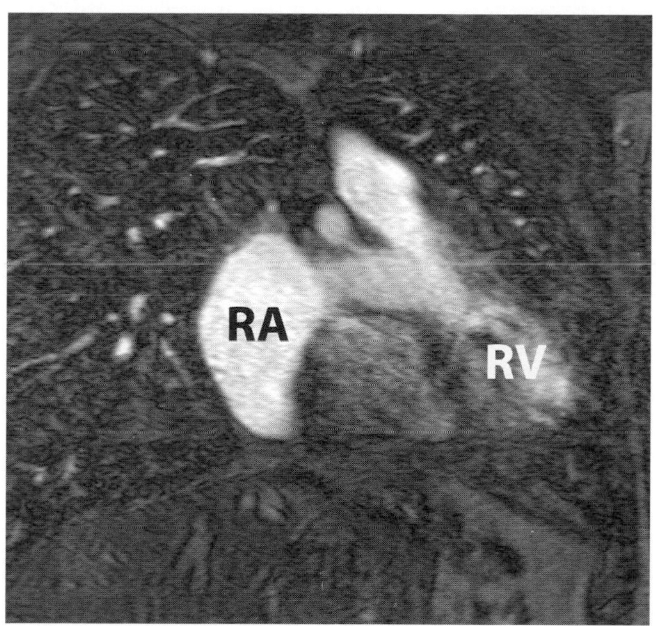

Coronal gadolinium-enhanced MR angiogram.

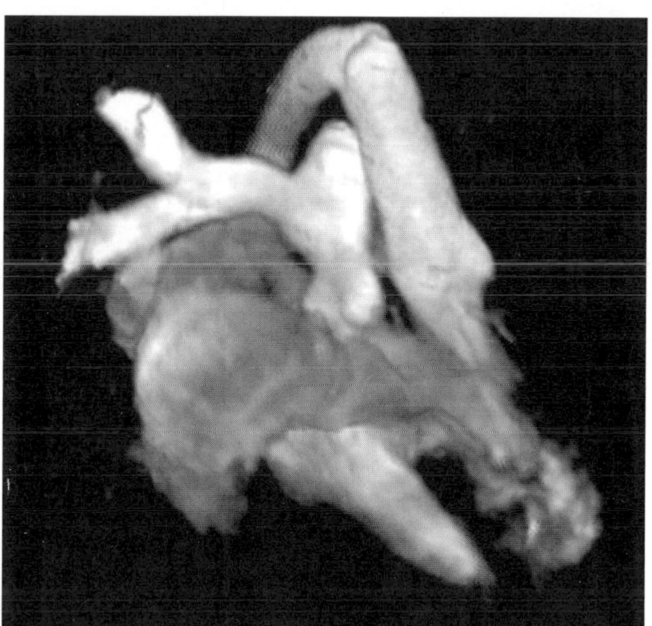

Volume-rendered gadolinium-enhanced MR angiogram.

1. Which great artery arises from the right ventricle?
2. Are the atrioventricular connections concordant or discordant?
3. Is the right ventricle on the right side or left side of the heart?
4. What is the diagnosis?

CASE 103

Inflammatory Constrictive Pericarditis

1. Marked thickening and enhancement.
2. Pericardium.
3. Inflammatory constrictive pericarditis.
4. Pericardial stripping.

Reference

Wang ZJ, Reddy GP, Gotway MB, Yeh BM, Hetts SW, Higgins CB. CT and MR imaging of pericardial disease. *Radiographics* 23(Special Issue)S167–S180, 2003.

Cross-Reference

Cardiac Imaging: THE REQUISITES, 2nd edition, pp 253–256.

Comment

Marked pericardial thickening and enhancement are seen in this child who had undergone repair of an atrial septal defect. In the presence of constrictive/restrictive physiology, the diagnosis is inflammatory constrictive pericarditis. If pericardial constriction were not present, the diagnosis would be acute pericarditis.

Constrictive pericarditis, whether acute or chronic, is treated by pericardial stripping.

Notes

CASE 104

Criss-cross Heart

1. The aorta.
2. Concordant. The right atrium connects to the right ventricle.
3. On the left side.
4. Criss-cross heart.

References

Nielsen JC, Parness IA. Anatomy of a criss-cross heart. *Circulation* 106:E41, 2002.

Araoz PA, Reddy GP, Thomson PD, Higgins CB. Images in cardiovascular medicine. Magnetic resonance angiography of criss-cross heart. *Circulation* 105:537–538, 2002.

Comment

Criss-cross heart is a rare anomaly in which the ventricular positions are transposed; this is known as an L-bulboventricular loop. The atrioventricular connections are concordant: the right atrium connects to the right ventricle and the left atrium connects to the left ventricle. The combination of concordant atrioventricular connections and the L-loop malpositioning of the ventricles creates long inflow tracts between the atria and ventricles. These tracts cross each other in a characteristic pattern that has been described on angiography. The tract between the right atrium and ventricle is seen in the image at the left.

This patient also has transposition of the great arteries.

Notes

CASE 105

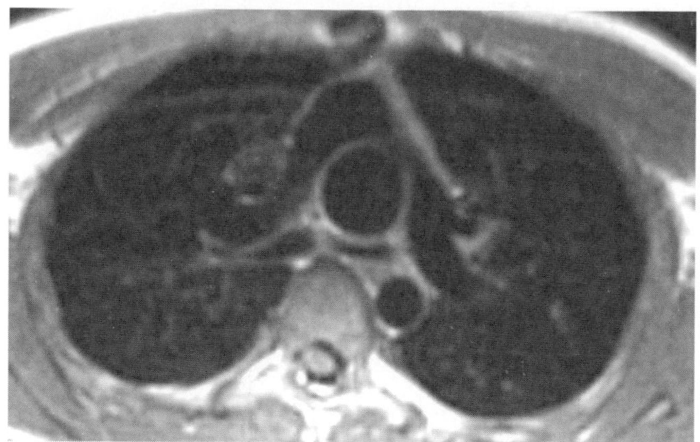

Axial spin-echo MR image.

1. Which operation was performed?
2. What was the original lesion?
3. Which complication has occurred?
4. What is the treatment?

CASE 106

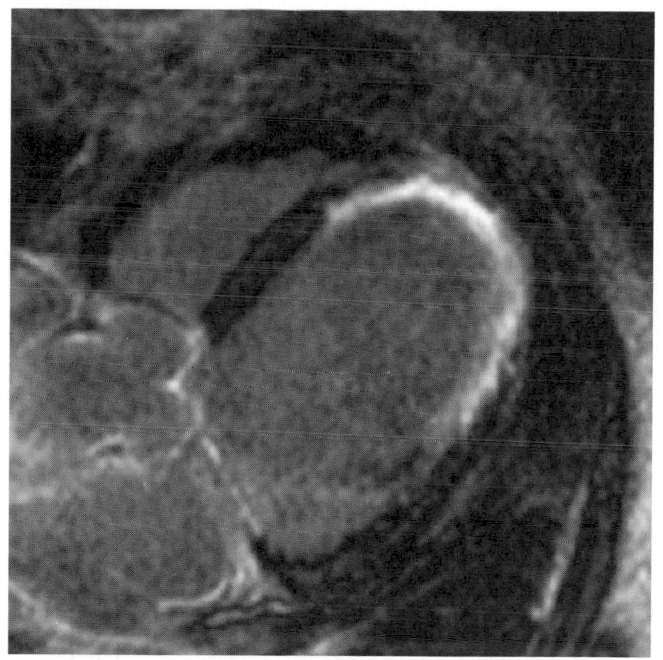

Long-axis delayed-enhancement MR image.

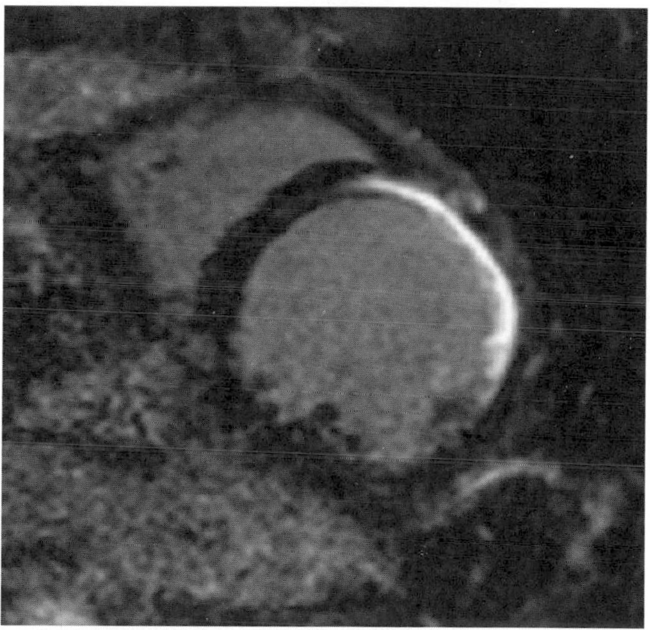

Short-axis delayed-enhancement MR image.

1. What type of imaging sequence is depicted?
2. Which abnormality is present?
3. What is the significance of this abnormal signal intensity?
4. What is the advantage of MRI over PET for this type of imaging?

CASE 105

Arterial Switch Procedure for Transposition of the Great Arteries, with Pulmonary Artery Compression

1. Jatene procedure (arterial switch).
2. Transposition of the great arteries.
3. Stenosis of the proximal left pulmonary artery.
4. Reoperation may be necessary.

Reference

Blakenberg F, Rhee J, Hardy C, Helton G, Higgins SS, Higgins CB. MRI vs echocardiography in the evaluation of the Jatene procedure. *J Comput Assist Tomogr* 18:749–754, 1994.

Cross-Reference

Cardiac Imaging: THE REQUISITES, 2nd edition, p 305.

Comment

For the past 15 years, arterial switch procedure has been the surgery of choice for repair of transposition of the great arteries. The pulmonary arteries are draped around the ascending aorta at surgery. One complication of the operation is stenosis of the central pulmonary arteries secondary to compression by the aorta. This condition may require reoperation.

Notes

CASE 106

Nonviable Myocardium

1. Delayed-enhancement MRI.
2. Hyperenhancement in the left ventricle.
3. It indicates nonviable myocardium.
4. The superior spatial resolution of MRI permits distinction of a zone of nonviability that is limited to the subendocardial region from transmural myocardial nonviability.

Reference

Pujadas S, Reddy GP, Lee JJ, Higgins CB. Magnetic resonance imaging in ischemic heart disease. *Semin Roentgenol* 38:320–329, 2003.

Cross-Reference

Cardiac Imaging: THE REQUISITES, 2nd edition, p 100.

Comment

The MR images show enhancement of the left ventricular apex and portions of the lateral and septal walls. The enhancing areas are not viable.

MR viability imaging is performed 7 to 10 minutes after intravenous administration of gadolinium chelate contrast medium. The myocardium enhances shortly after administration of the contrast agent, but the agent washes out of viable areas. Only nonviable myocardium enhances on the delayed images.

In a patient with impaired regional function in the left ventricle, determination of viability can be important for management decisions. A revascularization procedure such as balloon angioplasty or coronary artery bypass graft surgery can improve contractility in hypofunctioning but viable tissue. However, nonviable myocardium will not benefit from a revascularization procedure.

Revascularization may be of benefit if the area of nonviability involves less than 50% of the myocardial thickness; for example, if is limited to the subendocardial region. MRI can often distinguish whether the area of nonviability involves greater or less than 50% of the myocardial wall thickness, an advantage over PET in the determination of viability.

Notes

1 Mitral Regurgitation, 3–4
2 Atrial Septal Defect, 5–6
3 Pericardial Effusion, 7–8
4 Coarctation of the Aorta, 9–10
5 Pulmonary Edema, 11–12
6 Aortic Dissection, Stanford Type B, 13–14
7 Aortic Regurgitation—Marfan Syndrome, 13–14
8 Ventricular Septal Defect, 15–16
9 Aneurysm of Ascending Aorta—Annuloaortic Ectasia, 17–18
10 Left Ventricular Thrombus, 19–20
11 Aortic Stenosis, 19–20
12 Pectus Excavatum, 21–22
13 Left Aortic Arch with Aberrant Right Subclavian Artery, 23–24
14 Aortic Dissection—Stanford Type A, 25–26
15 Ruptured Aortic Aneurysm, 25–26
16 Prosthetic Heart Valves, 27–28
17 Left Ventricular True Aneurysm, 29–30
18 Calcific Pericarditis, 31–32
19 Mitral Stenosis, 33–34
20 Acute Traumatic Aortic Injury, 35–36
21 Tetralogy of Fallot, 37–38
22 Mitral Annular Calcification, 37–38
23 Right Aortic Arch with Aberrant Left Subclavian Artery, 39–40
24 Left Atrial Thrombus, 39–40
25 Coronary Artery Calcification, 41–42
26 Aortic Dissection—Stanford Type A with Pericardial Hemorrhage, 43–44
27 Pericardial Cyst, 45–46
28 Tricuspid Regurgitation, 49–50
29 Cardiac Angiosarcoma, 49–50
30 Superior Vena Cava Syndrome, 51–52
31 Traumatic Pseudoaneurysm of the Aorta—Chronic, 53–54
32 Persistent Left Superior Vena Cava, 55–56
33 Eisenmenger Syndrome: Atrial Septal Defect, 57–58
34 Left Ventricular False Aneurysm, 59–60
35 Periaortic Infection in Aortic Valve Infective Endocarditis, 59–60
36 Tetralogy of Fallot on MRI, 61–62
37 Large Left Ventricular True Aneurysm, 63–64
38 Left Atrial Myxoma, 65–66
39 Tetralogy of Fallot with Absent Pulmonary Valves, 67–68
40 Pseudocoarctation of the Aorta, 69–70
41 Congenital Pulmonary Valve Stenosis, 71–72
42 Aortic Arch Aneurysm, 73–74
43 Takayasu Arteritis, 75–76
44 Pacemaker in Patient with Persistent Left Superior Vena Cava, 77–78
45 Truncus Arteriosus, 79–80
46 Aneurysm of Coronary Artery Bypass Graft, 81–82
47 Constrictive Pericarditis, 83–84
48 Cardiac Lymphoma, 83–84
49 Pneumopericardium, 85–86
50 Intramural Hematoma—Stanford Type B, 85–86
51 Patent Ductus Arteriosus, 87–88
52 Dilated Cardiomyopathy, 87–88
53 Pericardial Metastasis, 89–90
54 Arrhthmogenic Right Ventricular Dysplasia, 89–90
55 Mitral Valve Prolapse, 91–92
56 Sinus of Valsalva Aneurysm, 91–92
57 Total Anomalous Pulmonary Venous Connecton—Type III (Connection below Diaphragm), 93–94
58 Hypertrophic Cardiomyopathy, 93–94
59 Double Aortic Arch, 95–96
60 Partial Anomalous Pulmonary Venous Connection, 97–98
61 Situs Inversus with Dextrocardia, 97–98
62 Mycotic Pseudoaneurysm, 99–100
63 Lipomatous Hypertrophy of Interatrial Septum, 101–102
64 Coronary Artery Stenosis, 101–102
65 Mirror-Image Right Aortic Arch, 103–104
66 Intramural Hematoma—Type A, 105–106
67 Pericardial Hematoma, 105–106
68 Pericardial Lymphoma, 107–108
69 Takayasu Arteritis—Long-Segment Coarctation of Aorta, 109–110
70 Anomalous Right Coronary Artery, 111–112
71 Complete Transposition of the Great Arteries, 113–114
72 Pericardial Lipoma, 115–116
73 Penetrating Aortic Ulcer, 115–116
74 Calcified Left Ventricular Aneurysm, 117–118
75 Pericardial Cyst, 117–118
76 Scimitar Syndrome, 119–120
77 Partial Congenital Absence of the Pericardium, 121–122
78 Pseudoaneurysm Secondary to Penetrating Ulcer, 123–124
79 Anomalous Left Coronary Artery, 125–126
80 Supracristal Ventricular Septal Defect, 129–130
81 Hypoplastic Left Heart Syndrome—Postoperative with Fontan Shunt, 131–132
82 Cervical Aortic Arch, 133–134
83 Hydropneumopericardium, 135–136
84 Pulmonary Atresia with Ventricular Septal Defect, 137–138
85 Interruption of Inferior Vena Cava with Azygous Continuation, 139–140
86 Cardiac Fibroma, 141–142
87 Ventricular Septal Defect, with Flow Measurements, 141–142
88 Pulmonary Regurgitation after Repair of Tetralogy of Fallot, 143–144
89 Coarctation of the Aorta, with Collateral Flow Measurements, 145–146
90 Effusive Constrictive Pericarditis, 147–148
91 Arrhythmogenic Right Ventricular Dysplasia with a Right Ventricular Aneurysm, 147–148
92 Pulmonary Sling, 149–150
93 Cardiac Hemangioma, 151–152
94 Hypertrophic Cardiomyopathy after Treatment, 153–154
95 Ebstein Anomaly, 155–156
96 Congenitally Corrected Transposition of the Great Arteries, 157–158
97 "Absent" Right Pulmonary Artery, 159–160
98 Myocardial Perfusion Defect, 159–160
99 Eisenmenger Syndrome Secondary to Cardiovascular Shunt—Aorticopulmonary Window, 161–162
100 Double-Outlet Right Ventricle, 163–164
101 Anomalous Left Coronary Artery Arising from Pulmonary Artery, 165–166
102 Interrupted Aortic Arch with Bypass Surgery, 167–168
103 Inflammatory Constrictive Pericarditis, 169–170
104 Criss-cross Heart, 169–170
105 Arterial Switch Procedure for Transposition of the Great Arteries, with Pulmonary Artery Compression, 171–172
106 Nonviable Myocardium, 171–172

A

Acute traumatic aortic injury (ATAI), 35–36
  pseudoaneurysm due to, 54
Aneurysm
  aortic
    ascending, 17–18
    pseudo-
      mycotic, 99–100
      secondary to penetrating ulcer, 123–124
      traumatic, 53–54
    ruptured, 25–26
  of aortic arch, 73–74
  of coronary artery bypass graft, 81–82
  of sinus of Valsalva, 91–92
  ventricular
    left
      calcified, 117–118
      false, 59–60
      true, 29–30
        large, 63–64
    right, arrhythmogenic right ventricular dysplasia with, 147–148
Angiosarcoma, cardiac, 49–50
Annuloaortic ectasia, 17–18
  in Marfan syndrome, 14
Anomalous left coronary artery, 125–126
  arising from pulmonary artery, 165–166
Aorta
  coarctation of, 10–11
    with collateral flow measurements, 145–146
    long-segment, 109–110
    pseudo-, 69–70
  overriding, 61–62
Aortic aneurysm
  ascending, 17–18
  pseudo-
    mycotic, 99–100
    secondary to penetrating ulcer, 123–124
    traumatic, 53–54
  ruptured, 25–26
Aortic arch
  aneurysm of, 73–74
  cervical, 133–134
  double, 95–96
  interrupted, after bypass surgery, 167–168
  left, with aberrant right subclavian artery, 23–24
  right
    with aberrant left subclavian artery, 39–40
    mirror-image, 103–104
Aortic dissection
  Stanford type A, 25–26
    with pericardial hemorrhage, 43–44
  Stanford type B, 13–14
Aortic injury, acute traumatic, 35–36
  pseudoaneurysm due to, 54
Aortic pseudoaneurysm
  mycotic, 99–100
  secondary to penetrating ulcer, 123–124
  traumatic, 53–54
Aortic regurgitation, in Marfan syndrome, 13–14
Aortic stenosis, 19–20
Aortic ulcer, 25–26
  penetrating, 115–116
    pseudoaneurysm secondary to, 123–124
Aortic valve
  bicuspid, 19–20
  infective endocarditis of, 59–60
Aorticopulmonary window, 161–162
Arrhythmogenic right ventricular dysplasia, 89–90
  with right ventricular aneurysm, 147–148
Arterial switch procedure, for transposition of the great arteries, with pulmonary artery compression, 171–172
Arteritis, Takayasu, 75–76
  with long-segment coarctation of aorta, 109–110
Ascending aorta, aneurysm of, 17–18
ATAI (acute traumatic aortic injury), 35–36
  pseudoaneurysm due to, 54
Atherosclerosis, 37–38
Atrial septal defect (ASD), 5–6
  with double-outlet right ventricle, 163–164
  Eisenmenger syndrome with, 57–58
  sinus venosus, 6, 97
Atrialization, of right ventricle, 156
Atrioventricular septal defect, 6
Autograft, 28
Azygous continuation, interruption of inferior vena cava with, 139–140

B

Barotrauma, pneumopericardium due to, 85–86
"Bat wing" pattern, 11–12
Bicuspid aortic valve, 19–20
Bioprosthesis, 28
Bridging vein, 55–56
Bypass surgery, interrupted aortic arch after, 167–168

C

Calcific pericarditis, 31–32
Calcification
  coronary artery, 41–42
  mitral annular, 37–38
Calcified left ventricular aneurysm, 117–118
Cardiac angiosarcoma, 49–50
Cardiac fibroma, 141–142
Cardiac hemangioma, 151–152
Cardiac lymphoma, 81–82
Cardiac neoplasms
  vs. left atrial thrombus, 40
  vs. left ventricular thrombus, 20
Cardiomyopathy
  dilated, 87–88
  hypertrophic, 93–94
    after treatment, 153–154
  restrictive, *vs.* constrictive pericarditis, 32, 82
Cardiovascular shunt, Eisenmenger syndrome secondary to, 161–162
"Cephalization," 12
Cervical aortic arch, 133–134
Coarctation of the aorta, 10–11
  with collateral flow measurements, 145–146
  long-segment, 109–110
  pseudo-, 69–70

Collateral flow measurements, coarctation of the aorta with, 145–146
Complete transposition of the great arteries, 113–114
Congenital pulmonary valve stenosis, 71–72
Congenitally corrected transposition of the great arteries, 157–158
Congestive heart failure, 11–12
Constrictive pericarditis, 32, 83–84
  effusive, 147–148
  inflammatory, 169–170
Coronary artery
  anomalous left, 125–126
    arising from pulmonary artery, 165–166
  anomalous right, 111–112
Coronary artery bypass graft, aneurysm of, 81–82
Coronary artery calcification, 41–42
Coronary artery stenosis, 101–102
Criss-cross heart, 169–170
Cyst, pericardial, 45–46, 117–118

D

Dextrocardia, situs inversus with, 97–98
Dilated cardiomyopathy, 87–88
Diverticulum of Kommerell, 24, 40
Double aortic arch, 95–96
Double-outlet right ventricle, 163–164
Doubly committed subarterial defect, 129–130
"Draped aorta" sign, 25–26
Ductus arteriosus, patent, 87–88
  after bypass surgery, 167–168

E

Ebstein anomaly, 155–156
  tricuspid regurgitation due to, 50, 156
Effusive constrictive pericarditis, 147–148
Eisenmenger syndrome
  with atrial septal defect, 57–58
  secondary to cardiovascular shunt, 161–162
Endocardial cushion defect, 6
Endocarditis, infective, of aortic valve, 59–60
Esophagopericardial fistula, 86
  hydropneumopericardium due to, 135–136
Ethanol septal ablation, for hypertrophic cardiomyopathy, 153–154

F

"Fat pad" sign, 8
Fibroma, cardiac, 141–142
"Figure 3" sign, 9–10
Fistula, esophagopericardial, 86
  hydropneumopericardium due to, 135–136
Flow measurements
  collateral, coarctation of the aorta with, 145–146
  ventricular septal defect with, 141–142
Fontan shunt, 131–132

G

Great arteries, transposition of
  arterial switch procedure for, with pulmonary artery compression, 171–172
  complete, 113–114
  congenitally corrected, 157–158
  with criss-cross heart, 169–170

H

HCM (hypertrophic cardiomyopathy), 93–94
  after treatment, 153–154
Heart valves, prosthetic, 27–28
Hemangioma, cardiac, 151–152
Hematoma
  due to acute traumatic aortic injury, 36
  with Fontan shunt, 131–132
  intramural
    Stanford type A, 105–106
    Stanford type B, 85–86
  pericardial, 105–106
  due to ruptured aortic aneurysm, 25–26
Hemorrhage, pericardial, Stanford type A aortic dissection with, 43–44
Heterograft, 28
Homograft, 28
Hydropneumopericardium, 135–136
Hypertrophic cardiomyopathy (HCM), 93–94
  after treatment, 153–154
Hypogenetic lung syndrome, 119–120
Hypoplastic left heart syndrome, 131–132

I

Immotile cilia syndrome, situs inversus and, 98
Infection, periaortic, in aortic valve infective endocarditis, 59–60
Infective endocarditis, of aortic valve, 59–60
Inferior vena cava, interruption of, with azygous continuation, 139–140
Inflammatory constrictive pericarditis, 169–170
Interatrial septum, lipomatous hypertrophy of, 101–102
Interrupted aortic arch, after bypass surgery, 167–168
Interruption of inferior vena cava, with azygous continuation, 139–140
Intramural hematoma
  Stanford type A, 105–106
  Stanford type B, 85–86

J

Jatene procedure, for transposition of the great arteries, with pulmonary artery compression, 171–172

K

Kartagener syndrome, situs inversus and, 98
Kerley B lines, 11–12

L

L-bulboventricular loop, 169–170
Left aortic arch, with aberrant right subclavian artery, 23–24
Left atrial myxoma, 65–66
Left atrial thrombus, 39–40
Left coronary artery, anomalous, 125–126
  arising from pulmonary artery, 165–166
Left subclavian artery, aberrant, right aortic arch with, 39–40
Left ventricular aneurysm, 29–30
  calcified, 117–118
  false, 59–60
  true, 29–30
    large, 63–64
Left ventricular failure, due to dilated cardiomyopathy, 88
Left ventricular thrombus, 19–20
Left-to-right shunt
  in aorticopulmonary window, 161–162
  in atrial septal defect, 5–6, 57–58
  in ventricular septal defect, 16
    with flow measurements, 141–142
    supracristal, 129–130
Lipoma, pericardial, 115–116
Lipomatous hypertrophy, of interatrial septum, 101–102
Lymphoma
  cardiac, 81–82
  pericardial, 107–108

M

Malignant neoplasm, pneumopericardium due to, 85–86
Marfan syndrome
  aortic regurgitation in, 13–14
  mitral valve prolapse due to, 91–92
Metastasis, pericardial, 89–90
Mirror-image right aortic arch, 103–104
Mitral annular calcification, 37–38
Mitral regurgitation, 3–4
Mitral stenosis, 33–34
Mitral valve prolapse, 91–92
Mycotic pseudoaneurysm, 99–100
Myocardial perfusion defect, 159–160
Myocardium, nonviable, 171–172
Myxoma, left atrial, 65–66

N

Neoplasms
  vs. left atrial thrombus, 40
  vs. left ventricular thrombus, 20
Nonviable myocardium, 171–172

O

Ostium primum atrial septal defect, 6
Ostium secundum atrial septal defect, 6
Overriding aorta, 61–62

P

Pacemaker, with persistent left superior vena cava, 77–78
Papillary muscle rupture, 3–4
Partial anomalous pulmonary venous connection (PAPVC), 6, 97–98
Patent ductus arteriosus, 87–88
  after bypass surgery, 167–168
Pectus excavatum, 21–22
Penetrating aortic ulcer, 115–116
  pseudoaneurysm secondary to, 123–124
Periaortic infection, in aortic valve infective endocarditis, 59–60
Pericardial cyst, 45–46, 117–118
Pericardial effusion, 7–8
Pericardial hematoma, 105–106
Pericardial hemorrhage, Stanford type A aortic dissection with, 43–44
Pericardial lipoma, 115–116
Pericardial lymphoma, 107–108
Pericardial metastasis, 89–90
Pericarditis
  calcific, 31–32
  constrictive, 32, 83–84
    effusive, 147–148
    inflammatory, 169–170
  tuberculous, 32
Pericardium, partial congenital absence of, 121–122
Persistent superior vena cava, 55–56
  left, with pacemaker, 77–78
Pneumopericardium, 85–86
Prosthetic heart valves, 27–28
Pseudoaneurysm, aortic
  mycotic, 99–100
  secondary to penetrating ulcer, 123–124
  traumatic, 53–54
Pseudocoarctation of the aorta, 69–70
Pseudotruncus, 137–138
Pulmonary artery
  "absent" (proximal interruption of) right, 159–160
  anomalous left coronary artery arising from, 165–166
Pulmonary artery compression, arterial switch procedure for transposition of the great arteries with, 171–172
Pulmonary atresia, with ventricular septal defect, 38, 137–138
Pulmonary edema, 11–12
Pulmonary regurgitation, after repair of tetralogy of Fallot, 143–144
Pulmonary sling, 149–150
Pulmonary valve(s), tetralogy of Fallot with absent, 67–68
Pulmonary valve stenosis, congenital, 71–72
Pulmonary venous connection, anomalous
  partial, 6, 97–98
  type III total, 93–94
Pulmonary vessels, enlarged, 11–12
Pulsus paradoxus, 7–8

R

Restrictive cardiomyopathy, *vs.* constrictive pericarditis, 32, 82
Rheumatic heart disease
  mitral stenosis due to, 34
  prosthetic heart valves for, 28
Rib notching, 10–11
Right aortic arch
  with aberrant right subclavian artery, 39–40
  mirror-image, 103–104
Right coronary artery, anomalous, 111–112
Right pulmonary artery, "absent" (proximal interruption of), 159–160
Right subclavian artery, aberrant, left aortic arch with, 23–24
Right ventricle
  atrialization of, 156
  double-outlet, 163–164
Right ventricular aneurysm, arrhythmogenic right ventricular dysplasia with, 147–148
Right ventricular dysplasia, arrhythmogenic, 89–90
  with right ventricular aneurysm, 147–148
Right-to-left shunt
  in Eisenmenger syndrome, 57–58, 161–162
  in tetralogy of Fallot, 38
Ruptured aortic aneurysm, 25–26

S

Scimitar syndrome, 119–120
Shunt vascularity
  in atrial septal defect, 5–6
  in ventricular septal defect, 15–16
Sinus of Valsalva aneurysm, 91–92
Sinus venosus atrial septal defect, 6, 97
Situs inversus, with dextrocardia, 97–98
"Snowman heart" appearance, 93–94
Stanford type A aortic dissection, 25–26
  with pericardial hemorrhage, 43–44
Stanford type A intramural hematoma, 105–106
Stanford type B aortic dissection, 13–14
Stanford type B intramural hematoma, 85–86
Subarterial defect, doubly committed, 129–130
Subclavian artery
  aberrant left, right aortic arch with, 39–40
  aberrant right, left aortic arch with, 23–24
Superior vena cava, persistent, 55–56
  left, with pacemaker, 77–78
Superior vena cava syndrome, 51–52
Supracristal ventricular septal defect, 129–130

T

Takayasu arteritis, 75–76
  with long-segment coarctation of aorta, 109–110
Tetralogy of Fallot, 37–38
  with absent pulmonary valves, 67–68
  mirror-image right aortic arch with, 104
  on MRI, 61–62
  pulmonary regurgitation after repair of, 143–144

Thrombus
left atrial, 39–40
left ventricular, 19–20
Total anomalous pulmonary venous connection, type III, 93–94
Transposition of the great arteries
arterial switch procedure for, with pulmonary artery compression, 171–172
complete, 113–114
congenitally corrected, 157–158
with criss-cross heart, 169–170
Traumatic aortic pseudoaneurysm, 53–54
Tricuspid regurgitation, 49–50, 156
Truncus arteriosus, 79–80
mirror-image right aortic arch with, 104
pseudo-, 137–138
Tuberculous pericarditis, 32
effusive constrictive, 147–148
"Tulip bulb" configuration, 18

U

Ulcer, aortic, 25–26
penetrating, 115–116
pseudoaneurysm secondary to, 123–124

V

Vasa vasorum, 105–106
rupture of, 86
Vascular ring
double aortic arch as, 96
pulmonary sling as, 149–150
right aortic arch with aberrant right subclavian artery as, 39–40
Vena cava
inferior, interruption of, with azygous continuation, 139–140
persistent superior, 55–56
left, with pacemaker, 77–78
Venolobar syndrome, 119–120
Ventricular aneurysm
left
false, 59–60
true, 29–30
large, 63–64
right, arrhythmogenic right ventricular dysplasia with, 147–148
Ventricular septal defect (VSD), 15–16
with double-outlet right ventricle, 163–164
with flow measurements, 141–142
pulmonary atresia with, 38, 137–138
supracristal, 129–130
with truncus arteriosus, 79–80
Vertical vein, persistent left superior vena cava *vs.*, 55–56

W

"Wall-to-wall heart"
in pericardial effusion, 7–8
in tricuspid regurgitation, 49–50
"Water bottle" configuration, 7–8